THE HEALTH CARE MANAGER'S HUMAN RESOURCES HANDBOOK

THE HEALTH CARE MANAGER'S HUMAN RESOURCES HANDBOOK

Charles R. McConnell

JONES AND BARTLETT PUBLISHERS
Sudbury, Massachusetts
BOSTON   TORONTO   LONDON   SINGAPORE

World Headquarters

Jones and Bartlett
Publishers
40 Tall Pine Drive
Sudbury, MA 01776
978-443-5000
info@jbpub.com
www.jbpub.com

Jones and Bartlett
Publishers Canada
6339 Ormindale Way
Mississauga, ON L5V 1J2
Canada

Jones and Bartlett
Publishers International
Barb House, Barb Mews
London W6 7PA
United Kingdom

Jones and Bartlett's books and products are available through most bookstores and online booksellers. To contact Jones and Bartlett Publishers directly, call 800-832-0034, fax 978-443-8000, or visit our website at www.jbpub.com.

Substantial discounts on bulk quantities of Jones and Bartlett's publications are available to corporations, professional associations, and other qualified organizations. For details and specific discount information, contact the special sales department at Jones and Bartlett via the above contact information or send an email to specialsales@jbpub.com.

ISBN-13: 978-0-7637-2597-6
ISBN-10: 0-7637-2597-8

Library of Congress Cataloging-in-Publication Data

McConnell, Charles R.
  The health care manager's human resources handbook / Charles R. McConnell.
    p. cm.
  Includes index.
  ISBN 1-56726-117-5
    1. Health facilities—Personnel management. 2. Personnel departments.
  I. Title.

RA971.35 .M2794 2003
361.1'068'3—dc21

2002035801

6048

Printed in the United States of America

10 09 08 07 06   10 9 8 7 6 5 4 3 2

About the Author

Charles R. McConnell retired following 18 years in health care human resources management with the affiliated organizations of ViaHealth, a multi-facility system based in Rochester, New York; 11 years as a senior consultant with the Management and Planning Services (MAPS) division of the Hospital Association of New York State (HANYS); and a prior career in industrial engineering. He is presently affiliated with The VMC Group, Niagara Falls, New York, as a management consultant and works as an independent human resources consultant as well. An active author and editor, he has published 13 books and some 250 articles and serves as the editor of a quarterly professional journal.

Mr. McConnell holds a BS in engineering and an MBA from the State University of New York at Buffalo.

Table of Contents

Preface

Most books written about human resources (HR) management present their information from the inside looking outward. That is, they use the language of human resources almost exclusively and are written primarily for human resources practitioners or students of human resources. Although any manager outside of a Human Resources department can acquire much useful information from them, these volumes are of most value to persons employed in HR capacities or preparing to become so employed.

The Health Care Manager's Human Resources Handbook is a somewhat different kind of book. Rather than presenting human resources topics and issues from the viewpoint of the practitioner, this book examines the field of human resources largely from the viewpoint of the department manager in a health care provider organization.

This is not another book written with the primary intent of telling its readers how the HR function operates in an organization. Although it necessarily contains a considerable amount of information that describes how HR operates, it is first and foremost a book that describes what the HR function can do for you, and it shows you how to get the most value out of a relationship with your organization's HR department. This book will guide you in accessing and using your organization's Human Resources capability to assist you in effectively managing your own organizational unit.

As an internal staff function or support activity, Human Resources does nothing to actively advance the creation of a product or to further the performance of a service for an organization's customers. However, Human Resources does exist to support and enhance the creation of products and the delivery of services. In the manner of any other staff activity, Human Resources has as the most broadly stated reason for its existence the support of the organization's primary activities. The organization can carry on to some extent without an HR function, but with an HR function the organization can carry on more efficiently and effectively than would otherwise be possible.

This book will not go into full detail about the inner workings of Human Resources, at least not to the extent that it would in addressing HR practitioners. Rather, for each topic presented, enough information will be provided to convey an understanding of what is done and why it is done. Then guidance will be offered concerning when, why, and how to best take advantage of certain HR services. Each topic will be presented in a way that provides an understanding of the reasons behind the processes applied by HR personnel and the positions that HR practitioners generally advocate. The level of detail of this information will vary as needed to provide that understanding.

For example, as a department manager you may require considerable detailed knowledge of what occurs within HR when disciplinary action is called for. You need to know the applicability of pertinent laws so you are able to avoid the numerous obstacles and pitfalls that plague the process, and you need detailed knowledge about progressive disciplinary processes because your job responsibilities require active involvement in applying them. For a number of other topics, such as performance appraisal, you also need detailed knowledge of HR's involvement to completely fulfill your departmental responsibilities.

For other topics, however, you need see only the tip of the iceberg of HR activity. One example is the Immigration Reform and Control Act (IRCA) of 1986. Although this particular piece of federal legislation raised many concerns and created additional and often frustrating work for Human Resources personnel, as a line manager your involvement with IRCA can be thoroughly addressed in a few brief paragraphs. Likewise, many of the details of some major aspects of benefits programs and their administration need not be of continuing concern to you. As long as you recognize and understand the portion of the iceberg that is visible to you, you need know little of the part that lies beneath the surface—except to know that it is there.

For most of the topics addressed in this book, four kinds of information will be presented:

- Some background information will be supplied to explain how certain topics came to be necessary or desirable parts of the HR responsibility. Because so much of what is done in Human Resources is governed by legislation, these explanations will include the legal rationale for the HR position or approach.
- The Human Resources responsibility will address what goes on within HR concerning some topics, and will provide whatever the manager ordinarily needs—detail if necessary, but only the tip of the iceberg if that is sufficient—to understand the Human Resources approach to the topic.
- Some information will address interfaces with line management, describing the outward appearance of some aspects of HR activity and identifying those points at which the HR department and the line organization meet at points of common interest and activity.
- Guidelines will be provided suggesting how you, the working department manager, can call upon the services of the HR department for maximum effect and benefit, so that you can get the best you can possibly obtain from your organization's Human Resources function.

A properly functioning HR department is a valuable resource for the organization. As with any resource, it should be used properly and to the fullest extent required—as efficiently and effectively as possible. Your organization's HR department exists to back you up as a manager, that is, to provide you with support and assistance in ensuring an interested, committed, well-functioning employee group.

If ever you believe you are not getting what you ought to be getting from your Human Resources department, put its staff on the spot. Challenge them. Reach out to help form the working relationship between Human Resources and line management that is so important to a well-functioning department. Let the information and guidance in this book show you how to encourage your Human Resources department to do the best it possibly can for you and your employees.

Charles R. McConnell
December 2002

PART I
Human Resources and the Organizational Environment

CHAPTER 1
From Employment Office to Human Resources

This chapter:

- Briefly reviews the history of Human Resources in business organizations, from a few scattered tasks to a centralized activity that, once established, began to take on additional tasks as they arose
- Establishes the rationale for having a Human Resources department
- Describes the mission of the Human Resources function in the organization.

AN EVOLVING FUNCTION

The Human Resources function (referred to throughout this work by the interchangeable terms Human Resources or simply HR) as it is known today originated and developed in the same manner as various other functions of the health care organization—or any other kind of organization for that matter. That is, it began with what we would now consider fairly narrowly defined responsibilities. Human Resources originated and grew in the same manner as Finance, Purchasing, and other functions. Bits and pieces of necessary work having some characteristics in common tended to be bundled or gathered together partly because they related to each other and partly because what they had in common suggested the need for certain skills and expertise. For example, activities that had to do with money—paying salaries, paying bills, receiving payments, maintaining bank accounts, handling investments—came together because they had financial matters in common. Thus, the finance function evolved, and the organization acquired a division or department known as Finance.

Before Human Resources there was Personnel, and in fact in some organizations the function remains known as Personnel. In some organizations the evolution from Personnel to Human Resources reflected real changes in overall scope and direction. Yet in many organizations the change occurred in name only, with the activity continuing unchanged in depth or breadth but with what to many had in recent decades become the preferred title.

And before there was Personnel there was the Employment Office.

Development of the Employment Office

Before the establishment of the Employment Office, individual managers did their own hiring. In many instances the organization was extremely small by today's standards, and the proprietor may have been the sole manager. As the business grew and the manager or managers became busier, they sought help, originally of a clerical nature, to assist with hiring.

The Employment Office came into being in some organizations because of the growth and accumulation of hiring-related tasks. There came to be enough work of this kind that it made sense to concentrate it in one place. No doubt one of the driving reasons for bringing these tasks together in one place was to relieve proprietors and managers of what had come to be regarded as a growing amount of work that did not contribute to turning out the organization's product or service but that had to be done so that the business could keep functioning.

The primary benefits of establishing the Employment Office were:

- Supervisors and managers were freed from having to find people to work
- The organization gained consistency in hiring practices.

Initially only two significant activities had to be carried out with regard to employees and their needs: they needed to be hired, and they needed to be paid. Before these activities became centralized both were usually accomplished by proprietors or their designees. In some instances the task of compensating employees became centralized before hiring did; various proprietors established the role of "paymaster." In many organizations the function of the paymaster was merged into the newly established Employment Office; thus, in this new function known as the Employment Office there were two primary activities that became known generally as Employment and Payroll.

The functions of Employment and Payroll grew in both scope and complexity as organizations were affected by legislation at all levels of their operations. With the introduction of wage and hour laws at both the state and federal levels and the advent of income and Social Security taxes, those who hired and paid employees began to assume increasing responsibilities within the business in addition to now having to answer to various government agencies.

Early in the twentieth century it was common for Employment and Payroll to be in the same organizational unit. In a few organizations Payroll remains part of Human Resources to this day, but in the overwhelming majority of organizations Payroll has long been part of Finance.

Tasks were added to the Employment Office as needs arose related to employees and the business of finding them, hiring them, and maintaining them as employees.

The label "Personnel department" began to attach itself to what had been the Employment Office, as it was far more descriptive of what the department's activities had become. The Personnel function, after all, dealt with many aspects of the organization's people.

The Expanding Personnel Function

Many employers responded to the forces of competition and other external pressures by beginning to offer forms of compensation other than wages. "Fringe benefits," as these added forms of compensation came to be called, required work on the part of the organization. The new tasks needed an organizational home, and since they related to employees—to people—the Personnel department was the natural place for them.

Along the way health insurance programs increasingly became part of many organizations' benefits offerings. Government mandates such as worker's compensation (originally called workmen's compensation) entered the picture as a statutory benefit. (Statutory benefits are benefits the employer is required by law to provide—the employer's share of Social Security taxes and participation in worker's compensation, unemployment insurance, and possibly state-mandated short-term disability). Retirement programs proliferated, also providing more work for the Personnel department.

A major piece of government legislation that caused a great deal of work for some organizations was the National Labor Relations Act of 1935, commonly known as the Wagner Act. This Act provided legal protection to labor unions and made it considerably easier than it had been for unions to organize workers. It also created a great deal of work for organizations that became subject to union organizing and that later had to function with a union in the conduct of their business. In many organizations, union-related activity, such as running an anti-organizing campaign or negotiating or administering a contract, devolved to those who were already in the "people" business. (Today, in an organization having unionized employees, an activity known as Labor Relations may exist on its own or as a function of Human Resources.)

Before the early 1960s the typical Personnel department was responsible for hiring employees, record keeping related to employees, some compensation and benefits administration, and possibly labor relations. Over the years leading up to the early 1960s the Personnel department developed an image of a staff or service group that ran an employment function, kept records, and generally pushed paper. In the early 1960s, however, the importance of the personnel function began to expand, and in 1964, with passage of the Civil Rights Act of 1964, the Personnel department was required to adopt a significantly expanded and increasingly important role. (See Chapter 3, The Legal Framework of Present-Day Human Resources, for a chronology of civil rights and human rights legislation.) The work of the Personnel department became increasingly complex, and the level of responsibility involved increased significantly. Much more specific knowledge was required of practitioners. Specialized education began to develop, and Personnel began to grow as a specific professional field.

Even as personnel work grew more complex, more requirements were placed on the function, more and different kinds of problems emerged, and more and different kinds of work had to be done, the former image of the Personnel department—those who find employees, keep files, and push paper—continued to prevail. Unfortunately, in many instances this old image was reinforced by personnel practitioners who, after perhaps two or more decades in the field, were overwhelmed by the tide of change and had fallen well behind the times.

In academia, personnel administration became a specialized educational field. Subdisciplines, some of them relatively narrow—compensation administration, benefits administration, testing and selection—began to arise.

In the mid-1970s, the personnel function became responsible for dealing with various external agencies and interest groups involved in interests such as affirmative action, equal employment opportunity, safety, and social responsibility.

Problems with "Personnel," Real and Perceived

Most of the personnel practitioners of the mid-twentieth century were not educationally prepared specifically for that field. When most of these practitioners received their education, education in personnel administration generally consisted of a course or two included in other programs.

Health care organizations, especially hospitals, were once viewed as—and in most instances in fact once were—low-pressure environments that offered escape for some who have been described, perhaps unfairly, as "industry dropouts." Many administrators, directors of finance, personnel managers, and others came into hospitals from various businesses and industries in mid-career. Some personnel managers, for example, left the manufacturing industry for hospital jobs as an escape from union involvement, which at the time was extremely limited in hospitals.

Some of the problems experienced with the "personnel" image, and some of the anti-personnel bias occasionally encountered, was surely due to the performance and behavior of personnel practitioners who found themselves in over their heads as the field became more complex and the pressures of the 1960s and 1970s continued to mount.

Many people who spend their entire working lives in one particular function do not readily adapt to change. Some of the practitioners of the old school—many of whom entered health care personnel work in the 1940s, 1950s, and early 1960s—fell by the wayside as the field became tougher and considerably more demanding. Some were unable to cope with unions and the demands of labor relations, some became frustrated by affirmative action and other civil rights concerns, and in the 1980s some gave up as increasing government regulation of benefits created a technical and legal quagmire.

There are still some undeniable image problems with the personnel function. Some managers still view the Personnel department as a minor staff function that does little more than hire people and file papers. Some employees view the function as a bureaucratic activity that is there primarily for the benefit of the corporation and not for them.

WHAT'S IN A (NEW) NAME?

Although today Human Resources is the prevailing name for the function, the label is far from universal in its usage. Many departments fulfilling the same overall function are still called Personnel departments, and some are known by other names as well.

Is "Human Resources" more descriptive than "Personnel"? Some contend that an organization's ultimate resource is financial, and the organization uses financial resources to acquire both things (material resources) and people (human resources). Therefore, in the organizational context "human resources" means "people"—as does "personnel."

Regardless of which name one prefers, it is not the name that makes the difference. What truly makes the difference is what the particular Human Resources department or Personnel department does, and how it does it.

Why the Change?

Personnel became Human Resources in many organizations for the following reasons:

- To reflect more appropriately what Personnel had become
- To improve the image and elevate the status of the function
- To enhance the professionalism of its practitioners.

Did Personnel become Human Resources to *escape* the image of Personnel? For some, the change was made more to overcome the outmoded view of Personnel and to gain acknowledgement and a measure of respectability.

A parallel image transformation occurred in finance, beginning with the original concept of bookkeeping, transitioning through accounting, and eventually becoming finance. This transformation is far from complete as far as image is concerned; witness how often we hear finance practitioners referred to as "number-crunchers" or "bean-counters." Also, ask any marketing professional what that field has gone through to escape stereotypes associated with the label *sales*.

Practitioners in every field are required to learn and grow; the alternative is to fall behind and eventually fail. In some occupational fields, however, change occurs more rapidly than in others. In Personnel—Human Resources—several bursts of change occurred within a brief enough period to represent the career spans of many practitioners.

Bias, whether real or perceived, cannot be overcome by a change of name. Nor can respectability be gained. Respect, however, can be earned over time as a new image develops—an image that has nothing to do with the function's name other than the minor advantage of having shed the tarnish that some associated with the Personnel name. Human Resources is taking its place among those activities viewed as essential in the present-day organization.

Here to Stay

For a number of years, Human Resources has been the growing name of choice for this function. The name has been adopted by professional organizations and publications formerly designated as serving "Personnel," a fairly good sign that the HR name will dominate.

The changeover of name was most evident during the 1980s. Surveys indicated that in 1986, some 40 percent of such departments used the Human Resources designation, but by 1990 the proportion was at 60 percent and still climbing. Also, the Human Resources title was more prevalent in larger organizations, in use in 80 percent or more of organizations having 2,500 or more employees.[1]

A number of additional surveys conducted during the 1980s and 1990s by professional HR organizations seemed focused primarily on the extent of the elevation of status through changes in function title (HR versus Personnel), job title of the top HR person (for example, Vice President versus Manager or Director), and at what level in the organization the function reports.

Where Human Resources is at present—or at least where it should be—is, first, changing to stay abreast of the health care organization's changing needs, and second, working constantly to transcend its traditional reactionary role and adopt a more proactive outlook. HR needs to be on hand to minimize undesirable occurrences through the systematic identification of potential problems, and then work to avoid them.

In addition to performing all the expected functions in support of the organization's employees, an up-to-the-present Human Resources department:

- Serves as a full-fledged partner on the administrative team

- Participates in strategic planning
- Guides succession planning for the organization
- Functions as an agent for necessary and healthy change.

Throughout the remainder of this book, the title Human Resources will be used as the prevailing name for the function. This use is not to be construed as claiming that any such department that may happen to be called Personnel or perhaps another name is any less than a legitimate Human Resources department. True differences do not reside in labels.

Discussion Points

1. Describe how you believe the business of locating, hiring, and maintaining employees was accomplished before the advent of an "employment office," including what activities were probably performed and who was likely to have performed them.
2. With specific reference to activities found in health care organizations, describe how three functions other than Human Resources might have evolved in a manner similar to the evolution of HR. In each instance describe the various activities that might have formed the basis of each activity as it is known today.
3. Describe what you believe to have been perceived as the primary benefits of gathering various employee-related activities together to form the "employment office."
4. Identify the two or three earliest changes that you believe influenced the development of a centralized activity to address matters related to employees. Why?
5. Explain why some consider the term "fringe benefits" to be misleading at best or completely erroneous at worst, and why the value of these benefits is most appropriately considered part of total compensation.
6. Comment on the "industry dropout" phenomenon regarding earlier full-time HR management in health care, explaining whether you believe the somewhat derogatory label is reasonably or unreasonably applied.

7. Develop an argument either for or against the continuing change of name from "Personnel" to "Human Resources" and prepare to defend your position in discussion with someone supporting the viewpoint opposite yours.

8. Develop an argument that either supports or opposes the abolition of a central personnel function in favor of having each individual manager look after all such activities for his or her own department.

9. Discuss whether you believe that changing the name of "Personnel" to "Human Resources" substantially improved the image of the function.

10. Comment on the following quotation from *Up the Organization* by Robert Townsend (Alfred A. Knopf, Inc., 1970): "Fire the whole personnel department. Unless your company is too large (in which case break it up into autonomous parts), have a one-girl people department (not personnel department)," keeping in mind that this passage was written in the late 1960s.

NOTES

[1]Dave Stier. "More Use of Human Resource Title," *Resource,* Society for Human Resource Management (SHRM), October 1989. p. 2. (SHRM was formerly ASPA, the American Society for Personnel Administration.)

CHAPTER 2

How Human Resources Fits into the Health Care Organization

This chapter—

- Provides an overview of the position of Human Resources within the organization
- Makes the distinction between line and staff activities and establishes HR as an essential staff function
- Describes a number of "models" of HR service delivery and perceived behavior
- Describes how the HR function is usually organized internally to serve the organization
- Considers the relationship between HR and executive management
- Introduces the relationship between HR and other departments
- Reviews HR's role in implementing change within the organization
- Reviews the effects of reengineering on human resources services
- Describes the trend toward "outsourcing" various HR services.

HUMAN RESOURCES IN THE ORGANIZATION: THE MACRO VIEW

In health care facilities the individual in charge of the Human Resources department will most likely report to one of the organization's two top executives: the President or Chief Executive Officer (CEO) or the Executive Vice President or Chief Operating Officer (COO). Most of today's health care Human Resources functions report to the top executive.

Human Resources will not ordinarily report to any level lower than the level that commands all operating line functions. For HR to report to a level other than executive management is inappropriate and impairs the function's potential effectiveness. Even reporting to the second executive level can at times result in conflict with other functions that report to the CEO. The COO normally has responsibility for all of the operating departments, including the overwhelming majority of employees, while certain other staff activities (e.g., Finance) report directly to the President or CEO. Instances can arise in which Finance and Human Resources are in disagreement, and if HR reports to the COO it can be perceived as "owned" by Operations and thus potentially incapable of fair and equitable dealings.

For the sake of maximum effectiveness in all organizational relationships, the individual in charge of Human Resources should report to the Chief Executive Officer.

LINE AND STAFF

Two distinctions are generally made in using the terms *line* and *staff*:

- What these two kinds of functions are and how they differ
- How authority, that is, the chain of command, applies to both but in somewhat different ways.

Doing versus Supporting

Simply defined, the difference between line and staff is as elementary as the difference between *doing* and *supporting*. Line functions actually perform the organization's work while staff functions make it possible to get the work done at all, and to get it done efficiently and effectively. One does while the other facilitates.

Another way to describe a line function is to say that it advances the work of the organization. In the manufacture of a physical product, for example, each line activity performed changes the state of the product and brings it closer to completion. In the provision of a service, each line activity performed advances the state of completion of the service. If a line function is ignored or otherwise omitted, the physical product is not finished or the service is not satisfactorily delivered. In the food service area of a hospital, for example, if one station on a tray assembly line is missing, the meals that are assembled on that line will be incomplete. As another example, if a nurse neglects to administer a particular medication when scheduled, the service to the affected patient is incomplete. When a line function does not occur, something important to the completion of the product or service does not get accomplished.

A staff function, on the other hand, does not advance the completion of the organization's work. Rather, it supports and enhances that work by making it possible to continue producing products or delivering services as intended. Remove a staff function from consideration and the productive work of the organization can still continue, at least for a time, but it may continue inefficiently, and it will eventually cease. Staff functions within a health care organization include, for example, Human Resources, Finance, Housekeeping, and Maintenance. None of these advance the provision of patient care, but if they are not performed then patient care will eventually experience inefficiencies and losses in quality. The primary role of staff functions is to maintain the service environment and capability, making it possible for line functions to continue.

In most instances it is possible to determine whether an activity is line or staff by imagining what would happen to the work flow if the activity were to cease. If a function is abandoned and the work flow is immediately disrupted, it is a line function. If there is no apparent short-term effect on work flow, it is a staff function.

What occurs when those engaged in line activities disagree with those who perform staff functions about how services should be provided or supported? If a conflict between line and staff cannot be resolved by the managers of the respective departments, it ordinarily goes to higher management.

The Chain of Command

The concept of line and staff can become somewhat confusing when considered in conjunction with the *chain of command.* In every department, whether line or staff, there is a chain of authority that runs from the department manager down through any subordinate supervisor and to the rank-and-file employees. Because of the chain of command that exists within a department, a manager of a staff activity is also a line manager, but within that function only. For example, the Director of Finance has line authority over the employees in Finance, but that authority does not extend beyond the boundaries of the department. So the Director of Finance can exercise authority within Finance but not outside Finance. Every staff function has within it this limited chain of command, which does not extend beyond the department. In line functions, however, the chain of command can extend down through several organizational levels; for example, the CEO has authority over the COO, who in turn has authority over the Director of Materials Management, who has authority over certain others, and so on to the final link in the chain of command. The chain of authority extends through all levels.

Occasionally a function seems to straddle the boundary between line and staff. One obvious example in a hospital setting is Dietary, which provides patient feeding and therapeutic dietetics—both line activities—and cafeteria and snack shop—both staff activities.

Human Resources is a staff function. The line and staff distinction is extremely important in considering where HR stands and how it operates. The manager in charge of Human Resources has line authority within Human Resources only. As a staff function, Human Resources has no authority over any employees outside its departmental boundaries. The HR department may be the organization's voice regarding personnel policy, compensation, benefits, and many of the legalities of employment, but it has no power of enforcement. Enforcement concerning HR matters and issues lies with line management and executive management.

Managers working in a health care organization need to understand that although Human Resources may report at or near the top of the organizational structure, it is a staff function, and its role is largely service and advisory. As such, HR has no authority over any other functions or departments in the organization. Human Resources is there to provide advice, guidance, assistance, and whatever other service may be needed and appropriate.

HUMAN RESOURCES MODELS

Human Resources may be viewed in a variety of ways depending on:

- Its placement in the organizational hierarchy
- Its image throughout the organization
- The behavior of HR management and staff
- The apparent organizational expectations of HR
- The traditional role of HR in the organization
- The demands placed on HR
- The education, training, and experience of HR staff.

The various perceptions of Human Resources can be viewed as models of HR service delivery. One approach advanced in the 1980s suggests that any of five models may be recognizable.[1] These are:

- Clerical model
- Counseling model
- Industrial relations model
- Control model
- Consulting model.

The Clerical Model

In some organizations the clerical model represents the long-held, and to some the unflattering stereotypical, view of "Personnel" as:

- Processors and filers of paper and keepers of records
- Trackers of various statistics and key dates
- Administrators of employee benefits plans.

Under the clerical model, the top manager of HR is likely to be experienced as a benefits administrator or have a similar practitioner orientation. In the organization where this model truly exists, Human Resources may rarely if ever be called upon to go beyond these expectations.

The Counseling Model

The counseling model is relatively common in hospitals or other service organizations where the total cost of employees represents a large portion of the budget, and where there is an emphasis on maintaining employees as effective producers. Under this model Human Resources is likely to:

- Function as an advocate for employees
- Function as a resource to managers for people problems, disputes, and disciplinary issues
- Place high priority on preserving privacy and confidentiality
- Actively stress training and development
- Lag somewhat in effective compensation and benefits administration
- Maintain a primarily reactive posture.

The Industrial Relations Model

The industrial relations model develops in organizations in which the work force is unionized, and there are periodic contract negotiations and considerable activity having to do with grievances and arbitrations. Under this model, HR functions specified by contract are performed automatically and as expected, with little room for flexibility or judgment in their performance. HR may be viewed as powerful within the organizational structure, but in a limited and not especially positive sense.

The Control Model

Observed in very few organizations, under the control model Human Resources holds substantial power, usually stemming from the charisma, personality, or individual strength of its top manager and key staff. The control-model HR department usually exerts control over any aspect of operations having HR implications. Consistent with this model:

* Little management action is taken without clearance by Human Resources
* The HR department is current and knowledgeable concerning all legal requirements
* Policies, procedures, and other work rules are thoroughly and consistently applied
* The Human Resources executive will be a key member of the organization's administrative team.

With this model in place, department managers may feel stifled and see the organization as inflexible, bureaucratic, and rule-bound. Under the control model, employee involvement activities receive minimal if any support.

The Consulting Model

The consulting model is usually found in larger organizations. Here the HR practitioners are usually expert resources, relied upon by employees, department managers, and executive management according to need. The services provided are determined by demand. However, this is primarily a *reactive* model that ordinarily has effective service going to the point of each apparent need but leaves some needs either unmet or unidentified.

These "models" roughly describe some dominant perceptions of Human Resources. We are unlikely to encounter any of these as pure types; what we encounter will usually be something of a mix of the characteristics of two or three models. However, in the *perceptions* of employees and their department managers, one particular model will prevail. Surely Human Resources is best used as more of a consultant or advisor and less as a clerical function.

The greatest single problem with all five models is that they are all primarily *reactive*. All of the HR services represented by the models are needed, and they should be delivered without any single model dominating or overwhelming. However, it falls to all of management—executive management, department management, HR management—to make Human Resources a true strategic partner.

ALTERNATIVE HUMAN RESOURCES MODELS

The late 1980s also saw the publication of another approach to "modeling" HR department functioning. The alternative models are in some ways similar to their original forms but suggest a somewhat different view. Using both lists of models should enable one to describe fairly accurately the delivery of HR services in any organization.[2] These alternative models are:

- Clerical model
- Legal model
- Financial model
- Managerial model
- Humanistic model
- Behavioral science model.

The (Alternative) Clerical Model

This is essentially the same as the basic clerical model. This model views HR's primary role as acquiring and maintaining reports, data, and records; performing routine tasks; handling paperwork; complying with regulations; and handling employment. This model presents HR as passive and relatively weak.

The Legal Model

In this model HR draws its primary strength from its expertise in legislation affecting employment. The human resources function operating in this model places most importance on compliance with all applicable laws, and may thus come to be viewed as something of a bureaucratic or occasionally obstructive function. Also, the legal model is frequently present when there is a union in place, consistent with the need to negotiate contracts, monitor contract compliance, and address grievances.

The Financial Model

A human resources function operating under the financial model displays maximum attention to human resources costs—in particular, indirect compensation costs such as health and dental insurance, life insurance, retirement plans, paid time off, and other benefits. Human resources practitioners working under this model frequently become well versed in matters of finance, often to the extent of holding financial matters in higher priority than employee relations matters.

The Managerial Model

Under the managerial model, HR practitioners often work within the bottom-line, productivity-oriented framework of the line managers, sharing the goals and values of line managers and making decisions accordingly. This model also lends itself to decentralization of HR services, under which line managers perform a number of HR functions. This model sometimes leads to inconsistency of HR practices (since certain practices are in many hands). Under this model HR has no particular strategic outlook or long-range planning involvement.

The Humanistic Model

The central idea of this model is that HR exists primarily to foster human values and potential within the organization. Individual employees are the primary focus of HR practitioners, and individual development and career planning are emphasized. Driving this model appears to be the belief that enhancing the work life of each individual enhances the effectiveness of the organization overall. The rising level of education and sophistication of employees in general and their expectations of high-quality work experience lend support to this model.

The Behavioral Science Model

This model assumes that the behavioral sciences (such as psychology, social psychology, sociology, and organizational behavior) provide the foundation for most HR activity. Indeed, this model is frequently applied to the design of performance appraisal systems, job evaluation systems, reward and incentive programs, employee development programs, and employee interest and attitude surveys. Increasing sophistication of both managers and employees provides some support for this approach.

As with the first set of "models," these recent alternative HR models are also unlikely to be found in pure form. There will always, for example, be strong perceptions of the existence of a clerical model, since HR, no matter how modern and sophisticated it becomes, will likely continue to do a significant amount of recordkeeping. And unless there is a marked reversal in the amount of legislation actively affecting employment—certainly unlikely—there will be times when a legal model appears to prevail. Nevertheless, for many HR departments one or two particular models will prevail, or at least seem to prevail according to the perceptions of line managers and rank-and-file employees.

THE HUMAN RESOURCES INTERNAL ORGANIZATION

The Human Resources department is customarily organized according to the organization's expectations of HR and essentially reflects the prevailing model.

Smaller organizations use HR generalists; larger organizations employ a mix of specialists and generalists. In larger health care organizations the specialists most often used (in descending order of the frequency with which they will most likely be encountered) are:

- Employment
- Compensation and benefits
- Employee relations
- Training and development
- Labor relations
- Equal employment opportunity (EEO)
- Security
- Safety.

Human Resources of course serves both internal customers (all employees at all organizational levels) and external customers (employment applicants).

HUMAN RESOURCES AND TOP MANAGEMENT

How Human Resources rates in the organization, how much real or perceived clout HR has, and the extent to which Human Resources is respected and involved, depends to a considerable extent on the CEO's attitude toward and expectations of HR.

Nearly all CEOs at a minimum want their Human Resources departments to perform recruitment, compensation and benefits administration, and personnel record keeping—essentially those activities ordinarily perceived as the nuts-and-bolts HR activities. There is of course much more to present-day Human Resources, but some CEOs want no more than this basic "personnel" function.

A considerable number of CEOs also expect their HR departments, primarily the HR managers, to serve as advisors on employee matters. In organizations where employees are unionized, the CEOs usually expect HR to monitor labor relations activities.

The occasional CEO wants a "don't-make-waves" Human Resources department that is essentially seen but not heard, one that will look after what are considered legitimate employee needs but not act as an advocate for innovation or positive change.

Some CEOs of course want a true, innovative Human Resources department. However, the number who simply say they want an innovative HR department is considerably larger than the number whose behavior demonstrates that they actually do want such an HR function.

What is expected of Human Resources is strongly influenced by the CEO's priorities. Very little can be expected to change if the top several organizational priorities are focused on simply "running the store." The executive who is so oriented tends to overlook HR's potential value in business and strategic planning, human resources planning, and the development of human resources strategies.

Some have theorized that as human resources-related tasks dramatically expanded in the 1960s, 1970s, and 1980s, Human Resources was so involved in keeping pace with demands, creating and updating necessary systems, and adding and expanding services, that as a discipline it missed an early chance to become a full partner in organizational management. Indeed it has long been a matter of debate whether Human Resources is a genuine planner and decision-maker or simply a firefighting activity.

It is of course important that executive management:

- Regard Human Resources as a professional specialty
- Take steps to ensure that HR is staffed and run by competent people who have been appropriately educated and trained
- Openly support the Human Resources department.

How does an evolving function that has long been considered a service of considerably less capability than it presently possesses become a strategic partner with its leader a full-fledged member of senior management? The field of Human Resources has been wrestling with this question for two or three decades without finding satisfactory answers. It has happened in some health care organizations, but in many this scenario has yet to become reality.

HR'S RELATIONSHIPS WITH OTHER DEPARTMENTS

From the departmental perspective Human Resources has traditionally been viewed as more administrative than advisory, more as a policy enforcer than a policy maker. Human Resources has traditionally been regarded as the "paper-pushers," hiring people and filing papers.

The proliferation of laws and regulations governing all areas of the employment relationship has been a major factor, perhaps the greatest factor, in the changing role and position of Human Resources. However, the managers of other departments often cannot see or do not appreciate the legal and regulatory obstacles that must be avoided; rather, they primarily see what appears to be a rule-bound bureaucratic function that all too often is trying to prevent them from doing something they feel they need to do. Even those who have a partial appreciation of HR's regulatory environment often come to view HR as little more than a necessary evil.

Many of the prevailing views of Human Resources prevent managers from seeking HR counsel or assistance until their needs have become critical. However, the time to call upon HR to help address a personnel problem that could lead to disciplinary action or perhaps even legal action is when the earliest signs appear, not when the issue becomes a full-blown problem.

If Human Resources is there to serve, why then is it still often viewed as an obstacle? Sometimes resistance comes about because of HR's approach and the attitude of its practitioners; when a function is perceived as a miniature bureaucracy, there are usually reasons for that perception in the behavior of HR staff. Also, often the reasons why Human Resources may offer recommendations contrary to what department managers want are not well communicated. Consider the following example.

A department manager has had a key position open for several weeks, and the lack of a person is making itself felt in the department's output and on the other staff who have been obliged to cover with overtime. An ideal candidate shows up, is referred to the manager by HR, interviewed, and immediately offered the position. This ideal candidate accepts and indicates the ability to begin work at any time. The manager's instruction to HR is: "I want this person to start work tomorrow."

However, HR's response to the manager calls for a delay. Say it is Monday or Tuesday when the person is interviewed; the recruiter in HR responds to the manager: "We have to have this person properly cleared. Even on a fast track the earliest starting date we can give you is next Monday." The manager understands that "properly cleared" means conducting reference checks and completing a pre-employment physical examination, but the manager insists on a next-day start and suggests that "The reference checks and the physical can be concluded next week, after the employee has been working a few days."

Human Resources refuses to sanction the immediate start, and the department manager proceeds to complain to other managers and perhaps up the line management chain of command about HR's inflexibility and unwillingness to cooperate. The involved HR representative stands firm, without appreciating that perhaps the department manager is unaware that regulations (at least in some states) legally prohibit a new employee starting work in a health care position before being medically cleared for work, or that the organization, reinforced by personnel policy, has an obligation to make a good-faith effort to check references before accepting an individual as an employee.

In this instance the HR representative is bound by state regulation and corporate personnel policy, but if the department manager is not aware of or does not fully understand these constraints, then HR's opposition will appear to be arbitrary resistance. It does little good for HR to cite policies and regulations to the manager; coming from HR such are often perceived as "more HR rules." What is required is the education of line management concerning those legal and regulatory restrictions on aspects of the employment relationship that have an impact on their activities.

It helps to remember at all times in dealing with Human Resources that HR does not command; rather, HR recommends. However, as in the example above, Human Resources has the responsibility not only to recommend for or against a specific action but to advise others of the possible consequences of that action.

A department manager should never expect HR to command and should avoid ever letting HR command by default. A defense for an unpopular action or decision that should never be heard up the chain of command in line management or by executive management is "This was really Personnel's decision," or "Human Resources made me do it." As a pure staff function, Human Resources operates by advising, counseling, suggesting, recommending, and perhaps by negotiating, persuading, or convincing, but never by commanding.

HEALTH CARE HR AND THE CHANGING SCENE

As with any other organizational activity, HR must change with the changing times. Both external and internal changes to the health care industry are affecting the ways in which health care is delivered and are thus affecting the provision of human resources services. The modern health care organization faces three kinds of change: technological, financial, and social. The three are of course interrelated, and these major areas of change have resulted in many specific changes in the ways in which health care is organized and delivered.

Technological change includes all advances being made in methods of diagnosis and treatment (e.g., all new or improved equipment, new procedures, new or improved drugs)—essentially all advances made in any dimension of restoring health and preserving life. But technological change collides with financial considerations as the costs of having the benefits of the latest and best available come into conflict with the pressures to stem the rapid increase of health care costs. And social change becomes a strong influence as we see the population aging and we experience the changing attitudes of today's generations.

The net results of the interplay of the three major categories of change have been manifested in a number of forces for change within the health care industry. Prominent among these are:

- Increasing financial pressure, as revenues are constrained from growing consistent with actual cost increases and in some instances are being reduced
- Increasing competition, as elements of a shrinking hospital system struggle to acquire or retain a share of available business
- Growing emphasis on outpatient care, with technological advances and financial pressures continually conspiring to move more modes of treatment to the outpatient setting
- The proliferation of free-standing specialty centers that perform some of the same services that hospital departments perform
- Active corporate restructuring, as provider organizations consummate mergers or other affiliations and form health systems
- An increasing turnover rate among health care executives, as some resign or are removed under mounting pressure while others discover that "merger-mania" results in fewer executive positions
- The increase of medical entrepreneurship, as individual providers establish specialties or attempt to tap specific market segments
- Growing emphasis on productivity (getting more output from the same or less input), as financial constraints and other shortages are felt
- Chronic shortages of certain critical caregiving staff, as various occupational and professional groups react to the combination of financial pressures restricting earning potential and the stresses of working short-staffed under increasing demands
- An increasingly better educated and more sophisticated workforce of employees who are far less likely than earlier generations to accept what they are offered without expressing what they want.

Change within the health care organization—or, for that matter, within any organization—occurs in one of two ways: either it is intentional, planned and executed for some specific purpose; or it is forced, coming about in response to circumstances beyond the organization's control. Health care organizations, and especially hospitals, experience far more reactionary change than planned change. This is probably because:

- Change is difficult to sell unless it is driven by crisis
- Not many organizations engage in planning that creates change
- Because of workload and continuing problems, top management seems to have little time to focus on change

- Resistance to change is usually pervasive throughout the organization
- Middle managers and department managers do not see themselves as agents of change
- Few members of management are skilled and effective at creating and managing change.

It can of course be suggested that every manager at every level should be an agent of change. In the Human Resources department it is especially important that there be a belief in fostering a climate conducive to constructive change, and that this belief be communicated in all of HR's dealings with managers and employees. Today's health care organization requires a culture of change that encourages innovation, rewards risk taking, and clearly values employee participation and input. Human Resources will best communicate its belief in the change process through:

- Up-to-date policies and procedures that convey respect for the capabilities of every employee
- Flexible job descriptions that allow room for innovation and employee participation and input
- A modern performance appraisal process that permits employees to set objectives for themselves and to participate in their growth and development
- A promotion and transfer system that makes real the espoused opportunity for growth and development
- A compensation structure that includes the opportunity to influence earnings through performance
- A flexible benefits structure that recognizes the divergence of individual needs encountered in the workforce.

Given its unique relationship to all line and staff functions and its mission to provide service for all employees, the Human Resources department is ideally positioned to be the health care organization's primary driver of internal change. Whether it is used as such is up to both executive management and HR's leadership.

HUMAN RESOURCES REENGINEERED

Reengineering is intended to make work processes easier and more productive. Although the term is often used to describe many improvement-oriented activities, it is considerably more involved than many realize. The term literally means *engineered again*. It involves addressing something that is currently being done and redesigning the process so that some objective is achieved—perhaps a saving in time, labor, or money, perhaps a reduction in materials and supplies consumed, or perhaps an improvement in quality without an increase in cost.

As applied to an entire organization or significant unit thereof, reengineering can de defined as *the systematic redesign of a business' core processes, starting with desired outcomes and establishing the most efficient possible processes to achieve those outcomes*.

At the heart of traditional methods-improvement or problem-solving processes is the way something is currently being done. These processes start with the current method and look for ways to eliminate steps or make improvements. By contrast, reengineering ignores—or *tries* to ignore, and therein lies a significant problem—how something is currently done, focusing instead on desired outcomes. As many who have been intimately involved in reengineering efforts have discovered, for someone familiar with the details of a current method it is practically impossible to ignore that method and not be influenced by some parts of it. Thus, process-oriented reengineering efforts are often actually method-improvement undertakings.

Reengineering as a business term has in many instances replaced a number of other "ings" that over the last couple of decades have included: reorganizing, downsizing, repositioning, rightsizing, revitalizing, and modernizing. The term reengineering has evolved as its intent has gradually been clarified, and it now connotes more of a focus on process and less on people. (Nonetheless, an announcement of impending "reengineering" has come to be synonymous with the likely loss of jobs.)

In Human Resources, reengineering consistently results in reductions of staff. Indeed, much HR reengineering has been undertaken specifically to reduce the cost of HR services, and surely reducing staff is one well-known way of reducing cost. In fact, Human Resources is so labor-intensive that, with the exception of reducing employee benefits, there is no way to remove significant cost from HR other than reducing staff. Driving most HR reengineering is major organizational change and the need to improve HR service, if at all possible, while reducing cost.

Effects of Reengineering on Human Resources Staffing

In the late 1980s Human Resources staff ratios in various areas of organizational activity were:[3]

- Finance organizations   1.5 HR staff per 100 employees
- Health care organizations   0.7 HR staff per 100 employees
- Manufacturing organizations   1.0 HR staff per 100 employees
- Median of all organizations   1.0 HR staff per 100 employees

Human Resources staff size in health care had fallen by more than 20 percent during the latter part of the 1980s, and it continued to drop during the 1990s, although at a somewhat lesser rate. At the end of the 1990s median HR staffing for all organizations remained at 1.0 staff per 100 employees while HR staffing in health care had softened to approximately 0.60–0.65 HR staff per 100 employees. At the time of this writing, several health care institutions informally sampled reported Human Resources staff ratios ranging from approximately 0.70 down to about 0.50 HR staff per 100 employees. It is clear that Human Resources staffs in many health care organizations have been reduced to a greater degree than the reductions in staff overall.

One negative effect of staff cuts resulting from reengineering (or just plain unadorned cost-cutting) is the reduction of some of the "soft" services of Human Resources, such as counseling employees. The "hard" side of HR—compensation, benefits, etc.—must be maintained out of necessity and in some instances consumes all or most of available HR staff. When there seems to be no one available to listen to their concerns, a few employees will turn to someone who *will* listen—perhaps an external advocacy agency or a labor union.

The Flatter Organization

Organizational flattening—the elimination of layers of management such that the institution's organization chart becomes "flatter"—often accompanies reengineering. As many managers discovered through the 1980s and 1990s, when an organization is flattened some "middle managers" are eliminated and the responsibilities of the remaining lower layer, usually the first-line managers or supervisors, are increased.

The typical Human Resources department, even in a mid-to-large health care organization, may have only three layers. The middle layer, usually the specialist-managers of activities such as employment, compensation, and benefits, may vanish, leaving only HR staff and an HR manager. When this occurs in an HR department, the organization's department managers must then relate directly with several staff-level individuals rather than with two or three specialist-managers.

Centralization versus Decentralization

Reengineering can lead to more centralization or decentralization as the organization seeks more cost-effective ways of getting the work done. Whichever occurs will affect not only HR personnel and how they do their jobs, but department managers as well.

When Human Resources activities are decentralized, individual managers will find it necessary to be much more aware of HR concerns because decisions must then be made closer to the organization's lowest levels. For example, if some aspects of Employment are decentralized, a department manager may have to screen incoming applications and decide which do or do not have the qualifications for a particular open position; HR would have assumed this responsibility before decentralization.

Certain forms of technology (e.g., computerized telephone systems) have led to the *centralization* of question-and-answer systems and other systems for geographically scattered organizations. For example, using some of the newer communication systems, employees at multiple locations have been able to transact business concerning their benefits without having to travel to an HR office. This in turn can make it possible for HR to maintain a smaller presence at satellite locations while handling all business of a particular type centrally. Also, for geographically dispersed organizations, toll-free numbers for employees who have benefits questions represent a partial replacement of HR staff with technology.

OUTSOURCING

"Outsourcing" can be defined as *having an external vendor provide, on a continuing basis, a service that would normally be provided within the organization.*"[4] Although outsourcing is frequently—some might say inevitably—linked to staff reductions in Human Resources departments, budget cuts and staff reductions are not always the leading reasons for turning to outsourcing. Exhibit 2-1 lists the reasons usually given for outsourcing.

Exhibit 2-1 Commonly Cited Reasons for Outsourcing Selected Human Resources Functions (From most frequently to least frequently cited)

- Take advantage of the expertise of specialists (e.g., pension plan administration, worker's compensation administration)
- Save staff time, and save time getting certain tasks accomplished
- Save administrative costs
- Allow staff to focus on needs more relevant to the organization's purposes
- Compensate for overload caused by increasing responsibilities
- Reduce Human Resources staff
- Make organizational and departmental budget cuts.

Cutbacks related to difficult economic times, plus reengineering and other efforts, have generated business for certain specialty firms as some organizations, including many hospitals and other health services organizations, have outsourced selected human resources activities. Exhibit 2-2 lists functions that are sometimes outsourced, along with the reasons for doing so.

The most commonly outsourced activity, although based in Finance more often than in Human Resources, is payroll. Payroll processing requires considerable detailed knowledge of the ins and outs of the Fair Labor Standards Act and related regulations having to do with payroll deductions and other aspects of payment. For example, simply determining what is known as the "regular rate" for payment of overtime premium can get complicated—included are regular earnings, shift differential premium, call-in payment but not necessarily on-call payment, and other considerations—and it is alarmingly easy to make mistakes in the process. Firms that specialize in payroll, however, have built all of the detail into automated payroll systems that fully account for all of the detailed requirements of wage payment. The client business need only submit the input information in the proper form at the proper time, and the payroll service creates the paychecks (or the direct deposits) and generates the necessary records. This particular form of outsourcing has relieved a great deal of frustration for businesses. In many instances it also saves money; some organizations, among them many smaller health care facilities, generate too little payroll work to justify paying a full-time pay-

Exhibit 2-2
Human Resources Functions Frequently Subject to Outsourcing

- Payroll (although it is noted that payroll is more often than not considered a Finance department function, much payroll input often flows through HR, and where payroll is accomplished—inside or outside—has an effect on HR staff).
- Outplacement services. Most organizations outsource this activity, as it is ordinarily an intermittent or infrequent need.
- Employee assistance program (EAP) administration. Most organizations that have EAPs outsource this activity, primarily to maintain employee confidentiality.
- Employee training and development. Many organizations contract with training specialists or consultants for training services, especially training that is provided intermittently (e.g., supervisory or management training).
- Relocation services. Relocation is often outsourced because the need for it is usually intermittent or infrequent.
- Benefits administration. Considerable benefits administration may be performed internally, but some is inevitably outsourced (e.g., pension plan administration, administration of various self-funded insurance programs such as dental, short-term disability, etc.).
- Compensation planning and administration. Some of this is occasionally outsourced, particularly executive incentive compensation plans.
- Recruitment and staffing. Some elements of this are sometimes outsourced. For example, an organization undergoing rapid expansion or the addition of a significant service may outsource the screening of applications and résumés as well as screening interviews and perhaps even employee selection for some positions.
- Candidate background checks. This activity is becoming more common in hiring for responsible and sensitive positions in health care. Very few organizations attempt to do their own background checks; this activity is nearly always outsourced.
- Safety and security. Relatively few organizations outsource these activities in their entirety, contracting with specialists to supply such services on a regular basis.

roll specialist or purchasing an automated payroll system, so the payroll service provider fills their needs.

Some downsizing of human resources functions has resulted in outsourcing to save money compared with maintaining staff to perform the functions. Human resources outsourcing has increased dramatically in the early part of the twenty-first century. It was reported in early 2002 that 74 percent of companies were outsourcing at least one HR function, up from 58 percent in 1999.[5]

Many small facilities lacking the resources to employ adequate full-time human resources staff rely heavily on outsourcing firms and professional employer organizations (PEOs), which essentially take over the human resources functions. When a facility contracts with a PEO its employees become co-employees of the PEO. The PEO charges a percentage of payroll (perhaps 2–4 percent) for its services, which usually includes benefits administration as well as payroll. In one specific instance, by contracting with a PEO, a medical practice having no more than 6 or 7 employees at most times reduced its costs of personnel administration from 9 percent of payroll to 3 percent of payroll.[6]

Reengineering aside, some Human Resources departments have outsourced certain activities for a variety of reasons. One reason of course is economic; some activities can be done at lower cost outside than is possible inside. Other activities, such as administering a self-funded health insurance or disability program and coordinating an employee assistance program (EAP), are often done outside for reasons of confidentiality—operating these programs internally would require that employees' personal and medical information be revealed to the employees administering the programs.

Additional outsourcing of Human Resources functions is often one of the results of reengineering. As HR staff are eliminated, adjustments are made in the HR workload. However, some essential tasks that remain may occur in such limited volume that it does not pay to retain and pay appropriately trained staff to perform them. The most commonly outsourced HR activities include insurance claim processing, EAP administration, retirement and savings plan administration, employee education, and employment candidate background checks.

EFFECTS ON CORPORATE CULTURE

Corporate culture comprises the shared basic assumptions and beliefs developed by an organization over time.[7] New employees can often tell in a relatively short time the "kind" of organization they have entered: high-pressure, laid-back, competitive, trustful, distrustful, or family-oriented, for example.

As it takes time for an organization's culture to develop to maturity, so does it take time for an organization's culture to adapt to change. Reengineering inevitably brings change, often considerable change.

For an organization's culture to accommodate change successfully, that change should ideally occur in increments that can be absorbed without trauma and at a pace that allows full assimilation of one significant change at a time. However, change affecting the health care industry has been so rapid that in many organizations there has been no chance for the corporate culture to resettle before it is once again thrown off balance.

Reengineering inevitably rocks the corporate culture, as do the other major forces that have been keeping the health care delivery environment in turmoil for two decades or longer: merger, acquisition, and other forms of affiliation; downsizing, rightsizing, and other forms of reorganization; increasing external regulation of health care; and all forms of cost-cutting and otherwise adjusting to the changing finances of health care.

Discussion Points

1. Describe in detail a specific "outsourcing" practice of which you are knowledgeable, and explain what you believe are the primary benefits achieved by having these services provided from outside rather than keeping them within the organization.
2. Thoroughly explain the principal shortcomings in a reporting relationship in which the chief Human Resources officer reports to any executive other than the Chief Executive Officer (CEO).
3. Explain the fundamental difference between a "line" activity and a "staff" activity and provide two clear examples of each in a health care setting.
4. Explain why can we say that a primary characteristic of "line" is also present within a clearly defined "staff" activity such as Human Resources or Finance.
5. Write a one- or two-sentence description of the organizational circumstances that could conceivably foster the appearance of each of the following "models" of Human Resources in a health care organization: clerical model; control model; industrial relations model; legal model; consulting model; financial model.
6. As viewed from your perspective as a department manager or prospective department manager, discuss which of the

Human Resources models appear to be most appropriate for managing personnel in a health care organization. Why?

7. Describe how the Human Resources function of a health care organization might evolve through multiple "models" as the organization grows and matures.

8. Explain, with a couple of hypothetical examples, how the expectations an organization's CEO holds concerning Human Resources can shape the "model" of Human Resources service delivery.

9. Identify what you believe are the primary areas of conflict between Human Resources and department managers. How might these be constructively addressed?

10. Cite several of the apparent advantages of the decentralization of Human Resources services, along with the potential risks associated with doing so.

11. Describe the results of organizational "flattening" and provide at least one example, either actual or hypothetical.

12. Identify the primary shortcoming of "reengineering" as it is pursued in modern organizations and explain why much of what is called "reengineering" is little more than refinement of existing practices.

NOTES

[1] Janet R. Andrews, "Is There a Crisis in the Personnel Department's Identity?" *Personnel Journal,* Vol. 65, No. 6, June 1986, pp. 86–93.

[2] Michael J. Driver, Robert E. Coffey, and David E. Bowen, "Where is HR Management Going?" *Personnel,* Vol. 33, No. 1, January 1988, pp. 28–31.

[3] Dave Stier, "More Use of Human Resource Title," *Resource,* Society for Human Resource Management (SHRM), October 1989, p. 2.

[4] Philip J. Harkins, Stephen M. Brown, and Russell Sullivan, "Shining New Light on a Growing Trend," *HR Magazine,* Vol. 40, No. 12, December 1995, p. 75.

[5] Knight Ridder News Service, "Outsourcing Human-Resource Tasks," *Democrat & Chronicle,* Rochester NY, February 17, 2002.

[6] Larry Perl, "Outsourcing, Health-Care Style," *Detroiter: For Business in Greater Detroit,* November 1996, p. 26.

[7] Robert J, Greene, "Culturally Compatible HR Strategies," *HR Magazine,* Vol. 40, No. 6, June 1995, p. 115.

CHAPTER 3

The Legal Framework of Present-Day Human Resources

This chapter—

- Describes the evolution of the regulated environment within which Human Resources must work in serving the health care organization
- Highlights 1964 as the pivotal year in which legislation affecting employment began to take effect, marking the onset of the government shifting considerable social responsibility to employers
- Includes a chronology of legislation affecting employment, beginning with the year 1932, with a brief explanation of each pertinent law
- Describes the cumulative effects of employment legislation to date.

A REGULATED ENVIRONMENT

This chapter provides a review of the laws affecting various aspects of the employment relationship. Each law is described in essentially non-legal terminology, focusing on its stated or apparent intent. Some of the effects of the more significant laws are considered, and in a few instances some apparently unintended effects are described.

The intent of this chapter is to provide sufficient background and knowledge of employment legislation so the department manager can develop an understanding of the impact of employment law on that role. An important disclaimer is in order at this point: Nothing in this chapter constitutes legal advice, and no such advice should be inferred from its contents. The manager with a question about the applicability of any particular point of law should take it to the appropriate people in the organization—perhaps Human Resources, Administration, or Risk Management—who can provide or obtain an answer.

The pivotal year when Human Resources (still called Personnel in most organizations) began to change was 1964, when sweeping civil rights legislation came into being. Title VII of the Civil Rights Act of 1964 marked the beginning of significant changes in relations between government and business, as well as a change in philosophy that would result in a completely new direction for government in its concern for its citizens.

Pre-1964: Regulation Minimal and Tolerable

Before 1964, businesses were free to deal with employees essentially as they chose, except for the requirements of wage-and-hour laws and labor-relations laws. Prior to 1964 the only laws that had a noticeable impact on the employment relationship were the Fair Labor Standards Act (FLSA) and related state laws, and the National Labor Relations Act (NLRA).

The Fair Labor Standards Act governed—and to this day continues to govern—payment of wages and other related conditions of employment. This and similar laws in some states are commonly referred to as *wage-and-hour laws.*

The National Labor Relations Act (and similar laws in some states), governing relationships between work organizations and labor unions, were relevant only to organizations where employees were unionized or where there was active union organizing.

Thus, pre-1964 there were few legal restrictions on how Human Resources could operate and how managers could manage. Most business organizations complied with the wage-and-hour laws as a matter of operating routine, and those organizations where there was a union presence, either organizing or by contract, generally complied with applicable labor laws.

The turning point of 1964 represented a change in philosophy concerning government's relationship with business. For years the governing philosophy had largely been one of "hands off" to the maximum practical extent; employers needed concern themselves only with wage-and-hour requirements and labor relations restrictions. But 1964 marked a significant change in the direction government would be taking on behalf of its citizens. Since 1964 government has been addressing many of the perceived needs of individuals by involving employers in meeting those needs. A brief chronology of the relevant laws follows.

Norris-LaGuardia Act (1932)

The first piece of legislation to significantly address the growing organized labor movement in the United States was the Norris-LaGuardia Act of 1932. This Act marked a significant shift in public policy concerning labor unions, from a posture of legal repression of unions and their activities to one of encouragement of union activity. Although the Act essentially legalized union organizing and affirmed workers' rights to organize for collective bargaining purposes, it did little to directly restrain employers in their conduct toward labor organizations. (During the first third of the twentieth century many workers who attempted to organize for collective bargaining lost their jobs because of their involvement, and sometimes their organizing efforts were countered with violence.)

Today the Norris-LaGuardia Act is not an active concern. It is mentioned here primarily as a point of information for its role as a fore-runner to labor legislation that followed in later years.

National Labor Relations Act (NLRA) (1935)

The National Labor Relations Act (also known as the Wagner Act) established a number of rules for the conduct of both unions and employers in labor organizing and collective bargaining situations. Although the NLRA seemed to favor unions and encourage their presence, it also set some boundaries on what unions could do in their organizing activities. In addition to affirming employees' right to organize, the NLRA made it illegal for an employer to simply refuse to deal with a union provided that the union had conducted a legal organizing campaign and had won a proper representation election.

The NLRA created the National Labor Relations Board (NLRB), the body charged with administering the Act by conducting representation elections to determine whether employees in particular groupings ("bargaining units") wished to have union representation.

The Act specified that a union chosen by the majority of the employees in an appropriate unit would be the exclusive representative of all the employees in the unit. Also, the NLRA specifically banned a number of management actions as constituting "unfair labor practices" (a term that surfaces frequently during union organizing activity).

The NLRA was later modified by the Taft-Hartley Act and the Landrum-Griffen Act.

Social Security Act (1935)

The Social Security Act established a basic system of contributory social insurance and a supplemental program for the low-income elderly. The system was expanded in 1939 to provide benefits to survivors of covered workers and dependents of retirees. Subsequently it was further expanded to cover workers who had become permanently disabled, and it was again expanded in 1965 to provide Medicare health insurance coverage for the elderly.

Fair Labor Standards Act (FLSA) (1938)

One dimension of the congressional intent of the Fair Labor Standards Act was to reduce the high unemployment rate that typified the years of the Great Depression by reducing work-week hours to a uniform standard, thus spreading available work over a greater number of workers. In addition to defining a "normal" work week, the FLSA set minimum pay rates, established rules and standards for the payment of overtime, and regulated the employment of minors. The FLSA remains the country's basic wage-and-hour law.

Labor Management Relations Act (1947)

This Act, popularly referred to as the Taft-Hartley Act, was an amendment to the National Labor Relations Act. The NLRA as passed in 1935 clearly favored unions over employers; the principal effect of Taft-Hartley was to "level the playing field" to some extent by more appropriately balancing the responsibilities and advantages of union and employer. Taft-Hartley also listed specific unfair labor practices. Although still viewed by many as a law favoring labor unions, Taft-Hartley was clearly a swing in the direction of management's rights.

Two points of immediate interest concerning Taft-Hartley:

- When we see or hear mention of the NLRA, the reference is to the NLRA *as amended by Taft-Hartley*.
- Taft-Hartley was itself amended in 1975 to specifically address not-for-profit hospitals by removing the exemption that had been in place under Taft-Hartley since its passage in 1947. The impact of these amendments is addressed in detail in Chapter 15, Avoiding—or Dealing With—a Union.

Labor-Management Reporting and Disclosure Act (1959)

Commonly known as the Landrum-Griffen Act, this was another amendment to the National Labor Relations Act. Since it amended the NLRA as amended by Taft-Hartley, it could perhaps be referred to as an amendment to an amendment. Among its numerous provisions, this Act required employers, including not-for-profit hospitals and other nonprofit health care facilities, to report in detail to the U.S. Secretary of Labor any financial arrangements or transactions that were intended to improve or retard the process of unionization. Various reporting and disclosure requirements were also placed on unions.

Equal Pay Act (1963)

The Equal Pay Act was actually an amendment to the Fair Labor Standards Act. It prohibited the payment of unequal wages for men and women who worked for the same employer in the same establishment for equal work on jobs requiring equal skill, effort, and responsibility and performed under similar working conditions. Simply put, people doing the same work in the same place in the same way had to be paid equally regardless of gender.

Although the Equal Pay Act came into being before 1964, it had no noticeable impact on the work of Human Resources and no effect on the department manager's role.

Title VII of the Civil Rights Act of 1964

With the enactment of this pivotal legislation, business in general experienced steadily increasing regulation of the employment relationship.

Title VII provided the legal basis for all people to pursue the work of their choosing and to advance in their chosen occupations subject to the limitations of only their individual qualifications, talents, and energies. This legislation defined unlawful employment discrimination as:

- The failure or refusal to hire an individual, or to discharge an individual, or to discriminate against any individual with respect to compensation or other terms, conditions, or privileges of employment because of that individual's race, color, religion, sex, or national origin
- Limiting, segregating, or classifying employees or applicants for employment in any way that would deprive them of employment

opportunities or otherwise adversely affect their status as employees because of race, color, religion, sex, or national origin.

The Civil Rights Act of 1964 also established the Equal Employment Opportunity Commission (EEOC) to enforce the anti-discrimination requirements of Title VII. (The Act was amended in later years to compensate for perceived erosion of its strength and effectiveness owing to a number of Supreme Court decisions.)

The Civil Rights Act of 1964 figures prominently in Chapter 7, How to Conduct a Legal—but Effective—Selection Interview, and at other points throughout this book.

Age Discrimination in Employment Act (ADEA) (1967)

The Age Discrimination in Employment Act legally established the basic right of individuals to be treated in employment on the basis of their ability to perform the job rather than on the basis of age-related stereotypes or artificial age limitations. The ADEA prohibits discrimination in employment on the basis of age in hiring, job retention, compensation, and all other terms, conditions, and privileges of employment.

Originally enforced by the Department of Labor (DOL), in 1978 enforcement of the ADEA was transferred to the EEOC. The threshold for defining age discrimination is 40; workers age 40 and older are a "protected class" for EEOC purposes.

The ADEA has had a direct effect on retirement. Before the ADEA, employers were free to mandate retirement at a specific age, most commonly 65. The ADEA raised the limit such that employers could no longer mandate retirement at any age younger than 70. When the ADEA was amended in 1986, the age 70 limitation was removed. Retirement could no longer be mandated by any specific age, and the sole legal criterion for continuing in one's employment was one's continued ability to do the job. (There are some exceptions under which retirement by a certain age can be mandated, such as for police officers, firefighters, airline pilots, surgeons, and certain policy-making executives.) In many instances the ADEA has enabled people who wished to keep working to do so, and thus has ensured the continuing employment of some workers who might otherwise have to depend on government assistance.

Occupational Safety and Health Administration (OSHA) (1970)

Created in 1970 and effective in 1971, OSHA represents highly influential legislation concerning employee safety in the workplace. The intent of Congress in establishing OSHA was to provide all employees with a workplace free from recognized hazards that are causing or can cause death or serious physical harm to employees. The Occupational Safety and Health Administration is authorized to promulgate legally enforceable workplace safety standards, respond to employee complaints, and make on-site inspections as necessary to follow up on employee safety complaints or on lost-workday injury rates that are considered excessive.

On May 25, 1986, OSHA began enforcing the second phase of an elaborate set of rules known formally as "Hazard Communication."[1] These rules provide workers the right to know what they are dealing with on the job in the way of hazardous substances. According to OSHA's hazard communication rules, health facilities are required to:

- Create programs for informing and training employees about hazardous substances in their workplace
- Ensure that warning labels on all incoming containers are intact and clearly readable
- Maintain copies of material safety data sheets (MSDSs) for all hazardous substances in the workplace
- Supply copies of MSDSs to employees upon request
- Maintain MSDSs in a current state, accessible to employees on all work shifts
- Inform and train employees in the nature and appropriate handling of hazardous substances at the time of initial assignment.

There are lists of more than 1,000 substances considered hazardous under OSHA regulations. In addition, a number of states now have "right to know" laws with similar requirements.

Generally, under federal and state standards for the handling of hazardous substances, employers must disseminate material data safety sheets, make certain that warning labels are always in evidence on workplace containers, and at all times be able to produce a written employee orientation program. It ordinarily falls to the department manager to ensure that these requirements are fully satisfied within the department.

Rehabilitation Act (1973)

Although disabled persons were mentioned in the Civil Rights Act of 1964, they were addressed separately for the first time in the Rehabilitation Act of 1973. The Act formally recognized that the handicapped were subject to cultural myths and prejudices similar to biases against women and ethnic minorities.[2] However, this law applied only to employees of the federal government and employers doing a certain amount of business with the government.

One portion of this Act prohibited discrimination in the hiring, promotion, and other employment of the handicapped, essentially paralleling Title VII of the Civil Rights Act of 1964. Another portion required employers doing more than $2,500 in business with the federal government to apply affirmative action in employing and promoting qualified handicapped individuals. Employers having more than 50 employees and fulfilling government contracts worth $50,000 or more were required to have written affirmative action programs per the requirements of the Office of Federal Contract Compliance Programs (OFCCP). Also required of employers was the "reasonable accommodation" of the physical or mental limitations of an employee or applicant.

The Rehabilitation Act is significant as a precursor of the Americans with Disabilities Act (1990).

Employee Retirement Income Security Act (ERISA) (1974)

ERISA established four basic requirements governing employee retirement plans:

- Employees must become eligible for retirement benefits after a reasonable length of service
- Adequate funds must be reserved to provide the benefits promised under the plan
- The persons who administer the plan and manage its funds must meet certain standards of conduct
- Sufficient information must be made available on a regular basis so it may be determined whether the ERISA requirements are being met.

This Act was later reinforced by legislation included in the Retirement Equity Act of 1984, which greatly increased the complexity of ERISA and added multiple layers of Internal Revenue Service (IRS) regulations.

Pregnancy Discrimination Act (1978)

The Pregnancy Discrimination Act determined that discrimination on the basis of pregnancy, childbirth, or related medical conditions was unlawful sex discrimination under Title VII of the Civil Rights Act of 1964. From this point forward, pregnancy has been considered a medical disability and is treated accordingly as a disability of 6–8 weeks' duration (length depending on whether federal or certain states' guidelines are applied).

Consolidated Omnibus Budget Reconciliation Act (COBRA) (1986)

This complex piece of legislation addressed many concerns; most pertinent to employment is that COBRA allowed for the extension of group insurance coverage to employees and their dependents on a self-pay basis for set periods of time (ranging up to 36 months maximum, depending on the "qualifying event," i.e., the reason for accessing COBRA), for those who would otherwise lose group health or dental coverage because of loss of employment, change in employment status, or certain other defined events. By making it possible for these employees and dependents to remain on the group contracts under which they had been covered, COBRA shifted to employers some of the cost of health coverage for many individuals who would otherwise be uninsurable except under government programs. As far as health insurance is concerned, COBRA is simply stopgap coverage; those who continue coverage under COBRA must secure other coverage after the eligibility period expires. Coverage can be continued up to 18 months for laid-off employees, 29 months for the disabled, and 36 months for dependents following separation, divorce, or the death of the employee. However, should the employer go out of business or for some other reason terminate its health insurance plan, rights under COBRA cease immediately.

Immigration Reform and Control Act (IRCA) (1986)

This Act required employers to review and as necessary modify their hiring practices, instituting procedures to verify that job applicants are either U.S. citizens or are otherwise legally authorized to work in the United States. This law established civil and criminal penalties for knowingly hiring, recruiting, referring, or retaining in employment persons designated as unauthorized aliens if so identified on or after November 6, 1986. The Act also prohibited employers from discriminating against job applicants on the basis of citizenship status or national origin.

Much initial business reaction to IRCA was strong, vocal, and negative. Because IRCA forces employers to take steps to screen out illegal immigrants—the majority of whom enter this country with employment as a goal—many believed that business was being made to perform a function that the government should be performing. For example, an early assessment of the Act declared: "This onerous piece of legislation for business turns every employer in the country, whether he or she hires a housekeeper or 10,000 auto workers, into an arm— an agent or a cop, if you will—of the Immigration and Naturalization Service (INS)."[3] Most employment legislation specifies the minimum size organization to which it applies; for example, the Family and Medical Leave Act (FMLA) applies only to employers of 50 or more employees. The Immigration Reform and Control Act pointedly applies to all employers of *one* or more employees, based on the premise that a significant number of undocumented aliens find work as household help.

This legislation has created work in the form of a verification document known as the "I-9 Form," which is ordinarily completed in Human Resources as part of the hiring process. The new employee or employee-to-be must furnish certain proofs of identity and, in the instance of legal aliens, proof of authorization to work in the United States. After examining (and usually copying) the appropriate documents, a representative of the employer signs the I-9 to attest to having seen those documents. The employer has three business days from the date of hire to get the I-9 Form completed. (If the term of hire is to be less than three days, the I-9 must be completed on the first day of employment.) Completed I-9 Forms are retained in employees' personnel files, where they are subject to audit by the Immigration and Naturalization Service. Financial penalties are imposed for missing or incomplete I-9s. Also, there can be significant legal repercussions should illegal aliens be discovered in the work force.

Some have claimed that the Immigration Reform and Control Act has resulted in increased employment discrimination. Employment applicants who look or sound foreign, especially Asians and Hispanics, are often faced with an increased likelihood of discrimination by employers who may shy away from hiring them because they fear inadvertently hiring illegal aliens and thus exposing themselves to action by the INS.

Pension Protection Act (1987)

This Act requires organizations with underfunded pension plans to make additional payments to the Pension Benefit Guarantee Corporation (PBGC), an agency established to guarantee benefit payments to participants of legally qualified defined-benefit pension plans. In addition to increasing employers' payments to the PBGC, this legislation reduces or eliminates the deduction of contributions by employers for better-funded plans.

The Drug-Free Workplace Act (1988)

The Drug-Free Workplace Act requires organizations having $25,000 or more in federal contracts or grants to make good-faith efforts to maintain a drug-free workplace and to establish drug education and awareness programs for employees. As a precondition to receiving a contract or grant, the law requires the organization to certify that it will provide and maintain a drug-free workplace. The manager of any department involved in any portion of a federal contract or grant will be involved at several points in the following process:

- The organization must notify all employees in writing (via a published statement) that the unlawful possession, use, manufacture, or distribution of a controlled substance is prohibited in the workplace. The statement must specify the penalties for violation.
- The organization must establish a drug-free awareness program to inform employees of: the dangers of drug abuse in the workplace; the external requirement of a drug-free workplace as a condition of contracts and grants; drug counseling, rehabilitation, or employee assistance programs that may be available to them; and the penalties to which the organization may be exposed for violations that occur in the workplace.

- The organization must require that each individual employee who is to be involved in the fulfillment of a contract or grant possess a copy of the organization's published statement concerning controlled substances.
- The organization must notify each employee receiving the controlled substances statement that he or she is expected to abide by all terms of the statement and to notify the employer of any criminal drug statute conviction for a violation in the workplace no later than 5 days after conviction.
- Within 10 days of receiving notice of such criminal drug statute conviction, the granting or contracting agency must be notified of the conviction.
- Within 30 days of receiving notice of an employee's criminal drug statute conviction, the employer must take appropriate disciplinary action against the employee or require the employee to satisfactorily complete an approved drug-abuse assistance or rehabilitation program.
- The employer must make a good-faith effort to maintain a drug-free workplace through implementation of the foregoing procedures.

All health care institutions have an interest in keeping the work environment free from the dangers to patients, visitors, and employees created by the use of illegal drugs or controlled substances. For a number of years the drug abuse problem in the workplace has made it necessary for employers to develop and implement various means of addressing this growing problem. Although the requirements of the Drug-Free Workplace Act apply only to employees engaged on federal contracts and grants, conscientious management suggests that a comprehensive policy and drug-free awareness program be implemented for all employees. Surely conscientious departmental management will have a strong interest in maintaining a drug-free work environment whether or not there are external requirements for doing so.

Employee Polygraph Protection Act (EPPA) (1988)

This legislation prevents most private-sector employers from requiring job applicants or current employees to take polygraph (lie detector) tests. Under EPPA, routine use of polygraph tests is permitted only in organizations that produce and distribute controlled substances, and those involved in nuclear power, transportation, currency, commodities, or proprietary information.

In most organizations an employee may be asked to submit to a polygraph when "other evidence" gives management reason to suspect an individual employee; we may hear this referred to as "reasonable suspicion" or, somewhat inaccurately, as "reasonable cause." However, an employee may not be disciplined or discharged based solely on the results of a polygraph test. Under EPPA the employer may not:

- Ask an employee or job applicant to submit to a polygraph test (other than in instances covered by the exceptions enumerated above)
- Take any adverse action against an employee or applicant for refusing to take a polygraph test
- Use, ask about, refer to, or initiate any adverse action based on a polygraph test an individual may have submitted to for a different reason (in other words, the results of a polygraph test a person has submitted to for one specific reason cannot be used for a different purpose).

Worker Adjustment and Retraining Notification Act (WARN) (1988)

This law requires employers with 100 or more employees at any individual site to provide advance notification of major reductions in force. The employer must provide 60 days' notice of an impending layoff of 50 or more employees, and must also notify local government and the state dislocated worker unit that provides employment and training services.

Americans with Disabilities Act (ADA) (1990)

This Act provides individuals with disabilities with the same protections afforded minorities and other protected classes under the Civil Rights Act of 1964, calling for access equal to that available to others in regard to:

- Employment
- Services and facilities available to the public, whether under private or public auspices
- Transportation
- Telecommunications.

Disabilities are broadly defined under the Act and include hearing and visual impairments, paraplegia and epilepsy, HIV or AIDS, and literally dozens if not hundreds of other conditions. The list of recognized disabilities is long, and it continues to expand as legal wrangling continues over what is or is not a disability.

The ADA prohibits employers from asking about a job applicant's medical conditions, if any, and imposing major limitations on pre-employment physical examinations. In actuality, a physical examination cannot be conducted until after a job offer has been extended. If a physical examination reveals a medical condition that does not affect the person's ability to perform the major functions of the job, the employer may be expected to make a "reasonable accommodation." The key to applicability of the ADA lies in an individual's ability to satisfactorily perform the "major functions" of a job; thus, an individual cannot be denied a job because an impairment prevents performance of a minor or non-essential activity. Thus, the employer may find it necessary to make a reasonable accommodation for the condition, provided that such accommodation does not cause unreasonable expense or hardship.

From time to time, the department manager may have reason to be familiar with some aspects of the law concerning disabilities. Involvement surely will come the manager's way should there have to be a "reasonable accommodation" for one or more employees in the department. However, it is not always possible to tell on sight whether an individual is disabled. Unlike race or gender, a disability may not be readily identifiable.

The manager need not be concerned unless he or she knows factually that a disability exists. To obtain the protection available under anti-discrimination laws, an employee must identify himself or herself as disabled; if a disability is neither apparent nor declared, the employee in question should be treated the same as any other employee. If as a manager you *suspect* the presence of a disability, but if one has not been declared, *do not ask the employee.* Moreover, do not give an employee unsolicited advice about some possible but undeclared problem; to do so is disparate treatment.

The Americans with Disabilities Act has been in the news frequently since its passage in 1990. Fully 10 years after its passage it was argued before the Supreme Court that the ADA went too far in allowing disabled public employees to sue state and local governments in federal court.[4] States and localities generally have immunity against such lawsuits unless Congress has documented sufficient discrimination to deny them that immunity and to invoke its power under the 14th Amendment to ensure that people have equal protection under the law. (Congress has never shown that the states were failing to enforce their disability laws.)

In a decision rendered in January 2002, the Supreme Court unanimously narrowed the number of people covered by the ADA. The opinion held that "[m]erely having an impairment does not make one disabled for purposes of the ADA"; that a person's ailment must extend beyond the workplace and affect everyday life; and that the ability to perform tasks that are of central importance to most people's daily lives must be "substantially limited" before an individual can qualify for coverage under the 1990 law.[5] In other words, the Court ruled that an individual who could function normally in daily living could not claim disability status because of physical problems that limited his or her ability to perform certain manual tasks on the job.

In another opinion that was viewed by some as a defeat for disabled workers, the Supreme Court ruled that disabled workers are not always entitled to premium assignments intended for more senior workers.[6] The practical implication of this ruling is that in the majority of instances seniority can take precedence over disability. Continuing its series of clarifications and rulings limiting rights under the ADA, in early June 2002 the Court ruled that disabled workers cannot demand jobs that would threaten their lives or health.[7] This arose from a case in which a worker with a particular medical condition wanted to return to his original position although it was considered medically risky for him to do so. The ADA's requirement for "reasonable accommodation" has always made exception for those who might be a threat to the health or safety of others on the job, but this most recent decision interpreted the exception as also applying to workers who may present a risk only to themselves.

Other cases are pending, and it is likely that the Americans with Disabilities Act will continue to be refined through Supreme Court decisions for at least the next few years.

Older Workers Benefit Protection Act (OWBPA) (1990)

This Act, amending the Age Discrimination in Employment Act (ADEA), clarified the authority of the ADEA relative to employee benefits. Although it required equal benefits for all workers, following a number of legal decisions the ADEA allowed reductions in benefits for older workers in instances where added costs were involved. The OWBPA removed the option for the employer to justify lower benefits for older workers and required that any waivers or releases of age discrimination must be voluntary, part of an understandable written agreement between employer and employee. In effect, this law says that an employer cannot unilaterally provide a reduced benefit to an employee on the basis of age.

Civil Rights Act of 1991

Amending the Civil Rights Act of 1964, the Civil Rights Act of 1991 allows employees to receive compensatory and punitive damages for violations committed with malice or reckless disregard for an individual's protected rights, and also allows women and disabled workers to sue for compensatory and punitive damages (a right they previously did not have). This Act also provides for jury trials in such discrimination cases; previously these were handled through non-jury processes. For employers the overall impact of this Act has been to increase the likelihood of longer and costlier legal processes and to increase potential penalties.

Family and Medical Leave Act (FMLA) (1993)

Applying to employers of 50 or more employees, FMLA permits eligible employees (those having been employed for at least one year and having worked at least 1,250 hours during the previous 12 months) to take up to 12 weeks of unpaid leave during any 12-month period when unable to work because of a serious health condition; to care for a child upon birth, adoption, or foster care; or to care for a spouse, parent, or child with a serious health condition. Under certain circumstances, leave may be taken intermittently or on some reduced leave schedule, potentially stretching any given leave over a period longer than 12 calendar weeks. Employees who are entitled to a certain amount of paid time off are ordinarily required to use that time as part of their 12 weeks, which most employees on leave ordinarily do rather than experiencing the entire leave without pay. The Family and Medical Leave Act does not take precedence over any state or local laws that provide greater leave rights.

While on approved leave, employees must continue to receive health care benefits but are not entitled to accrue vacation, sick time, or seniority. The employer must guarantee that upon returning from leave an employee will be reinstated to the previous position held or placed in a fully equivalent position with no loss of benefits.

In many instances the Family and Medical Leave Act has made life considerably more difficult for department managers. When an employee in an essential position takes leave, that position must be covered; some positions cannot be left vacant for a few days, let alone for a 12-week period. Filling the position and later returning the employee to "an equivalent position" is not readily accomplished; "equivalent" has repeatedly been interpreted by courts and other external agencies as essentially the same in all ways—pay, benefits, tasks, responsibilities, often even hours and shift. The strict interpretation of "equivalent" often makes the safest course of action the preservation of one's original position, so the manager is left to juggle coverage— perhaps with temporary employees, overtime, reassignments, and other means—until the employee returns from leave. The FMLA has thus made staffing and scheduling more difficult and time-consuming for some managers.

Retirement Protection Act (1994)

The Retirement Protection Act strengthens and accelerates funding of underfunded pension plans and increases Pension Benefit Guarantee Corporation (PBGC) premiums for plans that pose the greatest risk, improves the flow of pension-related information for workers, and increases PBGC's authority to enforce compliance with pension obligations.

Small Business Job Protection Act (1996)

Despite the name of this Act, its provisions are not applicable to small businesses only. This legislation includes the 1996 increase in the minimum wage. It also increases pension protection and makes it easier for workers to roll over their retirement savings upon changing employment. It also somewhat simplifies pension administration and reduces the vesting period for certain multi-employer plans from 10 years to 5 years. It also makes it possible for certain smaller employers to establish simplified 401(k) plans.

Health Insurance Portability and Accountability Act (HIPAA) (1996)

This Act allows workers to continue health benefits when they change employment or lose their jobs and eliminates the possibility that an employee can be denied coverage because of pre-existing medical conditions. It also requires insurance companies to provide coverage for small employer groups or to individual employees who lose their group coverage.

FOR THE ORGANIZATION: GREATER RESPONSIBILITY, INCREASED COST

The foregoing chronology is not complete. There are a variety of state laws to contend with, as well as other federal laws that have employment implications (as appropriate, their effects will be mentioned elsewhere in this book).

It is not difficult to conclude that the final two decades of the twentieth century saw government spreading its influence over an increasing number of aspects of the employment relationship. In addition to creating added work for Human Resources, many of these laws, in designating what cannot be done or what must be done, have proscribed boundaries within which management must manage.

The pattern of employment legislation during the late twentieth century, continuing into the twenty-first century, has been to make employers more socially responsible for their employees. This is especially evident in significant pieces of legislation such as the ADA and the FMLA. These laws affecting social responsibility, and most of the other pertinent laws, have added work and supporting systems to the organization and increased the cost of doing business—and thus increased costs to the ultimate consumers of all good and services.

Some new laws have required only minor changes in procedures or modest alterations in recordkeeping practices. However, most have clearly increased the cost of doing business because the provider organization, and eventually its customers, are the only ones available to pay. Legislators know very well that it usually costs *something* to implement a new law in the workplace (although the legislators and the organizations that must comply with the law are often far from agreement about *how much* it will cost to implement a new law). When legislators create a new program, they undoubtedly know there are but three ways available to pay for its implementation: (1) they can discontinue an existing program to free up some funds, but rarely does this happen because it is always a politically unpopular move; (2) they can raise taxes to pay for it, but this is even more politically unpopular; or (3) they can find someone else to pay for it. The "someone else" who has been paying to implement all these laws affecting the employment relationship is business and, eventually, the consumer.

A CUMULATIVE EFFECT

Exhibit 3-1 lists the laws discussed by decade of passage. It is not difficult to see the shift from the pre-1964 concern with collective bargaining and wage and hour issues to the growing post-1964 concern with social responsibility.

A simple comparison of the pre-1964 years with the present day should serve to demonstrate how significantly the employment environment has changed. Although a few of the laws replaced features of earlier legislation, most of the laws passed since 1964 have exerted new and often different influences on how work organizations treat employees and how managers can manage their departments. The accumulation of nearly four decades of legislation affecting the employment relationship has taken "Personnel" from the days of the Employment Office to the modern Human Resources department and has placed upon the department manager countless "rules" for managing employees. There is little doubt that the future will bring more regulation.

A new law can come into being in a relatively brief period of time, yet the changes in human behavior required by that law can be a long time happening. A strong case in point is Title VII of the Civil Rights Act of 1964. Employment discrimination has now been prohibited by law for the greater part of four decades, but problems of discrimination continue in many organizations. Nevertheless, the work force in the United States is becoming increasingly diverse, and only the organizations that eliminate discrimination will be able to properly value and manage this diversity.

For the greater part of four decades employee rights have been an extremely active legal topic in the federal and state legislatures and thus in the courts. We can expect this interest in individual rights to continue, probably even to intensify from time to time. The employment environment has changed and will continue changing; those who manage within this environment must either change with it or be left behind.

Exhibit 3-1 Employment Legislation by Decade

1930s
  Norris-LaGuardia Act (1932)
  National Labor Relations Act (1935)
  Social Security Act (1935)
  Fair Labor Standards Act (1938)
1940s
  Labor-Management Relations Act (Taft-Hartley) (1947)
1950s
  Labor-Management Reporting and Disclosure Act (1959)
1960s
  Equal Pay Act (1963)
  Title VII of the Civil Rights Act (1964)
  Age Discrimination in Employment Act (1967)
1970s
  Occupational Safety and Health Administration (OSHA) (1970)
  Rehabilitation Act (1973)
  Pregnancy Discrimination Act (1978)
1980s
  Consolidated Omnibus Budget Reconciliation Act (COBRA) (1986)
  Immigration Reform and Control Act (IRCA) (1986)
  Pension Protection Act (1987)
  Drug-Free Workplace Act (1988)
  Employee Polygraph Protection Act (1988)
  Worker Adjustment and Retraining Notification Act (1988)
1990s
  Americans With Disabilities Act (ADA) (1990)
  Older Workers Benefit Protection Act (OWBPA) (1990)
  Civil Rights Act of 1991
  Family and Medical Leave Act (FMLA) (1993)
  Retirement Protection Act (1994)
  Small Business Job Protection Act (1996)
  Health Insurance Portability and Accountability Act (HIPAA) (1996)

Discussion Points

1. Explain why 1964 and the passage of Title VII of the Civil Rights Act of 1964 are referred to as the turning point in the evolution of Human Resources. Other than 1964 representing the beginning of a steady flow of regulations, what is it that truly constituted a change of direction? Why?

2. Define and describe a "bargaining unit" as pertinent to present-day applicability of the National Labor Relations Act.
3. Review when and how the Equal Employment Opportunity Commission (EEOC) was established and what its purpose is.
4. Define a *bona fide occupational qualification* (BFOQ) and provide at least two specific examples.
5. Explain what the "right to know" laws primarily address and what they are intended to accomplish.
6. Well before the passage of the Americans With Disabilities Act (ADA) certain employers were required in some instances to provide "reasonable accommodation" of the limitations of an employee or applicant. Specify when this occurred and enumerate the conditions under which this requirement applied.
7. Identify the primary intended purpose of the Employee Retirement Income Security Act (ERISA). Explain why this legislation was likely seen as necessary.
8. Discuss the principal business effects of the Immigration Reform and Control Act (IRCA).
9. Pose two hypothetical examples of situations in which a health care employer might legally require a polygraph (lie detector) test as a condition of either initial employment or continued employment.
10. View the Family and Medical Leave Act (FMLA) from the perspective of a working department manager and describe the ways in which this legislation has affected the manager's ability to manage.

NOTES

[1] Bruce D. May, "Hazardous Substances: OSHA Mandates the Right to Know," *Personnel Journal,* Vol. 65, No. 8, August 1986, p. 128.

[2] Steven Fox, "Employment Provisions of the Rehabilitation Act," *Personnel Journal,* Vol. 66, No. 10, October 1987. p. 132.

[3] Roger Skrentny, "Immigration Reform—What Cost to Business?" *Personnel Journal,* Vol. 66, No. 10, October 1987, p. 53.

[4] Hearst News Service, "High Court Scrutinizes Disabilities Act," *Democrat & Chronicle,* Rochester NY, October 12, 2000.

[5]Newsday, "High Court Limits Disability Law," *Democrat & Chronicle,* Rochester NY, January 9, 2002.

[6]The Associated Press, "Seniority Outweighs Disability, Court Says," *Democrat & Chronicle,* Rochester NY, April 30, 2002.

[7]The Associated Press, "Top Court Disallows Dangerous Jobs for Disabled," *Democrat & Chronicle,* Rochester NY, June 11, 2002.

PART II
The Health Care Manager Meets Human Resources

CHAPTER 4

Human Resources and the Health Care Manager

This chapter—

- Briefly describes the functions that are part of Human Resources—almost always, often, and occasionally
- Provides an alternative breakdown of Human Resources services by overall functions—acquiring, maintaining, retaining, and separating employees
- Identifies the activities for which the department manager can expect contact and involvement with Human Resources, and the likely extent of that contact and involvement
- Compares and contrasts line management and Human Resources management in terms of background and perspective as well as other characteristics for the purpose of explaining some of the tensions that sometimes develop
- Sets the stage for eventually overcoming the apparent differences between Human Resources and line management.

HUMAN RESOURCES FUNCTIONS

All Human Resources departments are pursuing essentially the same overall mission—providing service to the organization and its employees—but not all HR departments are organized in the same fashion and not all perform all of the same functions. In certain organizations some functions that are often associated with Human Resources may be performed by other departments or may even be departments in their own right.

In the sections that follow we will consider a three-level division of Human Resources functions:

- Those that are commonly associated with HR and are usually part of the HR department
- Those that are often but not always part of the HR department
- Those that are occasionally associated with Human Resources or sometimes found within the HR department structure.

Usually Active Human Resources Department Functions

The first three of the following functions are invariably part of Human Resources, and the fourth is usually part of HR if there is a union present in the organization.

Employment or Recruitment

This activity addresses the original function of what we previously described as the "employment office." It may go by different names here and there, but *employment* or *recruitment* is usually part of the function's organizational designation.

This is of course the activity concerned with finding prospective employees, screening them, and scheduling them for interview by various supervisors and managers; extending official offers of employment; and performing a number of other tasks that are necessary to bring new hires into the organization.

With a diminishing number of exceptions, employment for the entire health care organization is centralized in Human Resources. The few exceptions that may still be found, especially in medium to large hospitals, usually involve nursing departments that continue to do their own recruiting. (This was formerly a much more common practice, although some nursing departments still maintain a "nurse recruiter" who works closely with Human Resources.) Also, it is relatively common for physician recruiting to be done elsewhere than HR, often from the office of the institution's medical director.

Compensation and Benefits Administration

Depending on the organization's size and mode of operation, "compensation" and "benefits" may be combined as a single activity or may be pursued separately by individuals who specialize in each. This latter situation is often the case in larger organizations.

The "benefits" portion of this activity was the next significant activity after "employment" to come into its own as a Human Resources function. The benefits activity ordinarily includes: explaining benefits to employees; answering benefits questions and assisting employees in accessing their benefits; maintaining relationships with certain benefits providers such as insurance carriers; keeping current with regulations that concern benefits; maintaining employee benefits records; and participating in the periodic assessment of the appropriateness of benefits (and when necessary becoming involved in designing and implementing benefits changes).

The compensation activity is of course concerned with wages and salaries, and its primary activities are ordinarily concerned with: recommending starting pay for new hires consistent with education and experience and the compensation of existing employees; addressing wage and salary questions and recommending corrective action when necessary; monitoring the organization's wage structure to ensure pay equity throughout the organization; and recommending changes in the wage structure consistent with pay changes in the community, the industry, and individual occupations as necessary.

Employee Relations

An activity such as employee relations is sometimes referred to as residing on the "soft side" of Human Resources. As opposed to the "hard side," primarily compensation and benefits, which deal largely with elements that can be quantified using dollars and cents and other numbers, the "soft side" addresses relations with people. An employee relations practitioner is likely to be involved, for example, in: advising supervisors and managers how to proceed in addressing certain employee problems; monitoring applications of the organization's disciplinary process; listening to troubled employees and referring them to sources of assistance as necessary; counseling individual employees as needs arise; serving as an employee advocate when necessary; and representing the organization in relations with external advocacy agencies such as the state division of human rights (or whatever it may be called in any particular state).

Labor Relations

Labor relations will exist as a separately identified function in larger organizations only if some or all of an organization's nonmanagerial employees are unionized. In a smaller setting, even with a union present there may not be enough continuing activity to justify labor relations as a separate function. When this is the case, the labor relations function often becomes part of another Human Resources practitioner's job, for example, an employee relations specialist or perhaps the Human Resources director.

Labor relations includes essentially what its name implies—continuing relations with the union or unions representing some or all of the organization's eligible employees. Much labor relations activity consists of: hearing and resolving complaints; processing grievances and representing the employer in related matters such as arbitration hearings and other formal processes; being actively involved in preventive labor relations when additional union organizing occurs; and participating in contract negotiations or related activity when necessary.

Often Human Resources Functions

Depending on the size of a particular institution and the way in which it is organized and how its activities are distributed, some of the following may exist as departments in their own right, as separately delineated functions within Human Resources, or as simply a few duties incorporated into the job descriptions of some of the HR practitioners.

Employee Health and Safety

Employee health may be in one spot organizationally and safety may be in another, or these activities may be combined. Either or both may report within Human Resources or within another departmental arrangement; for example, employee health may be part of Human Resources, or it may be part of one of the organization's medical divisions. It is not uncommon to find employee health as a sub-function of HR reporting to the chief HR officer, the rationale being that employee health is a service to employees and is thus serving "personnel," and that employee health also performs pre-employment physical examinations and is thus related to HR's employment section.

Training and Development

Training and development is often a sub-function of Human Resources but is also frequently found, again depending much on organizational size, as a separate, free-standing function reporting to another major department. One fairly common arrangement is for training and development to be attached to the nursing department (which may go by some more broadly encompassing name such as "patient care services"). Because of long-standing in-service education requirements, the nursing department often had an organized education function well before other departments' educational needs began to be recognized. As a result, training and development was long the province of nursing alone, and in many places it remains so, with education provided from there but across departmental lines.

Training and development will sometimes be split, with education of a clinical nature remaining with the nursing department and other education, such as nonclinical skill training and management development, falling under the chief Human Resources officer.

Security

The security department is ordinarily a fairly self-contained department, except in very small organizations where it may be among the functions of, for example, plant maintenance or building services. As a distinctly separate security department with a manager of its own, it may be one of the functions reporting to the chief Human Resources officer, or it may just as likely report within the plant facilities chain of command or to the administrator who oversees general services.

Child Care

If the health care organization operates a child care center or child care program, it is about equally likely that the individual who manages child care will report either to the chief Human Resources officer or to another person such as the administrator for general services. Since a child care center is subject to unique state licensing arrangements governing staffing and facilities, it usually appears as a distinctly separate entity. The rationale for attaching it to Human Resources is, again, the service-to-employees character of the activity. There are, however, differences in how health care organizations having child care programs define their scope of service—some limit themselves exclusively to an employee clientele, but many are open to the community. (The practice of some child care programs is to give priority to employees, but after meeting employees' needs to fill remaining capacity from the community.)

Award and Recognition Programs

Responsibility for award and recognition programs will ordinarily be part of another activity's responsibility rather than a separate entity (except in an extremely large organizational setting such as a large teaching institution that is part of a university and thus is served by the parent organization's award and recognition function).

In the majority of health care organizations, award and recognition programs are the responsibility of Human Resources, often falling to an employee relations practitioner. In some organizations, however, such programs are the responsibility of the public relations or community relations function, and perhaps occasionally administration.

Equal Employment Opportunity/Affirmative Action

If equal employment opportunity (EEO) or affirmative action exists as one or two named functions within the organization, they will usually be under the Human Resources umbrella. The person designated responsible for EEO, ordinarily an employee relations practitioner or Human Resources executive, has the primary responsibility for monitoring the organization's compliance with all applicable anti-discrimination laws. The individual in this position will also be charged with some of the responsibilities that fall under employee relations, particularly those relating to external advocacy agencies such as the state division of human rights and the Equal Employment Opportunity Commission (EEOC).

Since affirmative action programs are no longer an active mandate, they are no longer an active pursuit in Human Resources. Affirmative action required organizations doing a certain amount of business with the government to demonstrate that positive efforts were being made to bring the composition of the work force into line with the composition of the organization's labor market area. In other words, the goal of an affirmative action program was to achieve a work force in which the percentage of women and minorities mirrored the percentage of women and minorities in the labor market area. When such programs were prevalent, they were commonly monitored by the individual responsible for EEO.

Occasionally Human Resources Functions

The following activities will sometimes be found within the Human Resources structure.

Risk Management

These days most health care organizations of any appreciable size have a risk management function. Risk management will include monitoring malpractice and liability actions brought against the organization, overseeing and constantly evaluating various insurance coverages, studying loss trends (such as costs under worker's compensation), and literally attempting to manage risk—to achieve an appropriate balance between certain costs of doing business and the potential exposure to various legal risks.

Although formerly a function of Human Resources in some organizations, risk management is today usually found elsewhere in the administrative structure. With its increasingly significant legal implications, risk management is frequently handled by in-house legal counsel; if it is a one- or two-person department in its own right, its manager will often have a legal background.

Executive Compensation Administration

If executive management is not included in the organization's payroll system—where it *is* in most instances—it is likely to be accomplished through an external confidential payroll service. Executive compensation is almost certain to be accomplished externally if the organization's top executives are under individual contracts or their compensation arrangements include incentive compensation. In any case, it is rarely directly in the hands of Human Resources but is more likely taken care of at the executive level within the finance function.

Organizational Development

In some organizations "organizational development" is little more than management development under a different name. Certainly attention must be given to the educational activities necessary to keep managers current with developments in health care as well as to help them cope with the changing times. True organizational development, however, goes beyond management development in that it encompasses the changing requirements of the organization itself, addressing the ongoing question: How should this organization be changing in philosophy, mission, and vision, and even in its organizational structure to meet the demands wrought by changing social and economic times and the changing health care delivery environment?

In addressing overall organizational needs, a comprehensive approach to organizational development will also include succession planning. Succession planning complements management development and in an important sense expands upon it, preparing managers at all levels not only to keep up but potentially to move up. This facet of organizational development emphasizes internal development of management talent. A comprehensive approach to organizational development will also include some means of identifying and educating potential supervisors and managers from among the rank-and-file employees.

If it exists as a separately identified activity—which occurs in a minority of health care organizations—it is usually found within the Human Resources structure reporting to the chief Human Resources officer in parallel with employment, compensation and benefits, and other HR functions. On rare occasions organizational development may be found in parallel with Human Resources itself, with its head reporting to the same executive as the chief Human Resources officer.

Employee Assistance Program

Ordinarily described as an employee benefit, an employee assistance program (EAP) is intended to assist employees in addressing certain personal problems that can affect their work performance. Primarily a referral program (that is, one that helps in identifying an individual's needs and gets the person pointed toward obtaining help), a capably functioning EAP can help control absenteeism, tardiness, and other circumstances that can affect job performance, while enhancing quality and productivity. Such programs commonly address alcohol and drug abuse, family and marital difficulties, legal and financial problems, compulsive gambling, and other personal problems.

The overwhelming majority of health care organizations have employee assistance programs. The EAP's "home base" within the organization is ordinarily Human Resources or employee health (which may itself be part of Human Resources). However, only occasionally is the EAP actually operated from within the organization. The EAP is usually coordinated by a contracted external provider, enabling employees to use this resource with the assurance that no one within the organization need know their personal problems. The Human Resources role is limited to simply putting an employee who expresses a need in touch with the external EAP coordinator.

Outplacement Services

Outplacement involves assisting displaced employees in finding new employment. Since outplacement services are offered and provided only in instances of reductions in the work force or elimination of specific management positions, outplacement will likely never exist as a permanent sub-function of Human Resources or any other organizational element. However, "outplacement" occasionally occurs when someone in Human Resources or elsewhere in the organization is able to assist a displaced employee in becoming situated with another employer.

Payroll

The payroll function was once a common adjunct to the "employment" activity of early "personnel" departments in many organizations; originally the only such needs with regard to employees were to hire them and to pay them. As years went by, however, payroll requirements became increasingly complicated, and the organization's finance functions became increasingly sophisticated; as a result, payroll tended to be relocated organizationally.

Payroll is still attached to Human Resources in some organizations, but these instances are few and becoming steadily fewer. Today most payroll activities are performed in one of two places. In most organizations that do their own payroll processing, the payroll function is part of the finance department (although another department, perhaps data processing or information systems, which may or may not also be part of finance, will be involved in running checks and reports). Many other organizations, especially those of small to medium size, use external contractors who specialize in payroll services. When outside payroll services are used, the input information from which they work will be submitted to them by the finance department (usually) or by Human Resources (occasionally).

These functions are summarized in Exhibit 4-1, Human Resources Department Organization: Functions Included.

What about "Outsourcing"?

Mentioned in Chapter 2 as a sometime consequence of reengineering, "outsourcing" is the business term used to describe the circumstances of having some function that was formerly done within the organization performed by an outside party. A business might consider outsourcing for any of several reasons:

Exhibit 4-1   Human Resources Department Functions

Usually Part of Human Resources
- Employment or recruitment
- Compensation and benefits administration
- Employee relations
- Labor relations (if union presence)

Often Part of Human Resources
- Employee health and safety
- Training and development
- Security
- Child care
- Award and recognition programs
- Equal employment opportunity/affirmative action

Occasionally Part of Human Resources
- Risk management
- Executive compensation administration
- Organizational development
- Employee assistance program
- Outplacement services
- Payroll

- The work to be done requires special skill or expertise, and there is not enough of it to justify hiring a skilled person to do it (for example, managing pension fund investments).
- The task requires expensive equipment, but there is insufficient work to justify purchasing that equipment (for example, printing a multi-colored, slick-paper annual report).
- By virtue of specialization or sophistication, an outside supplier may be able to perform the task more economically (for example, performing outplacement for displaced executives).
- Staff reductions have created some "orphan" functions, i.e., tasks that must be done but for which time is unavailable to the remaining staff.
- A particular function occurs irregularly and takes insufficient time to justify training and retaining someone to do it (for example, publishing an employee newsletter).
- The work is of a sufficiently sensitive nature that confidentiality is best served by going outside (for example, coordinating an employee assistance program).

The decision to outsource any particular task will ordinarily involve considerations of cost, capability, and confidentiality. Also, many outplacement decisions are driven by staff reductions resulting from reengineering or straightforward downsizing. Often when a decision is made to eliminate a position, much of that position's work may be eliminated, modified, or combined with the work of another; however, certain essentials that remain to be done may be outsourced.

Of the Human Resources functions enumerated in this chapter, the activity most likely to be outsourced is outplacement services, which is a somewhat specialized activity that may be required only occasionally. Next most likely to be outsourced is the employee assistance program, largely for reasons of employee privacy and confidentiality. The next most likely to be outsourced is pension plan administration, followed in most instances by the administration of worker's compensation and disability programs.

A national survey of hospitals' HR services conducted in the late 1990s concluded that the only activity that is apparently more subject to outsourcing than Human Resources is legal services.

Another Breakdown of Human Resources Functions

Human Resources functions are often grouped into four major functions:

- Acquiring employees
- Maintaining employees
- Retaining employees
- Separating employees.

Exhibit 4-2 lists these four major functional groupings and the activities that usually fall within them.

Acquiring Employees

This category of activity includes everything that is undertaken to find employees and bring them into the organization—all employment or recruitment activity, including job fairs, recruiting trips, employment advertising, pre-employment testing, checking references and verifying credentials, new employee orientation, and in general any activity undertaken to acquire employees and get them initially situated in their positions.

Exhibit 4-2   Human Resources Activities by Major Functions

Acquiring Employees, including:
- Employment (recruitment): All activities that are part of or directly related to finding employees and bringing them into the organization.

Maintaining Employees, including:
- Compensation administration
- Benefits administration
- Personnel policies and procedures
- Performance appraisal programs
- Personnel record keeping
- Employee assistance program
- Employee health service
- Education and development
- Parking
- Cafeteria
- Communication programs
- Savings and investment programs.

Retaining Employees, including:
Many of the same mechanisms of "maintaining" employees can be cited as helpful in employee retention. Certainly pay levels and benefits in general are both maintenance and retention factors, as are the presence of education and development opportunities, performance appraisal programs, and employee assistance programs. Other specific retention strategies may include:
- Retirement plans
- Award and recognition programs
- Child care assistance
- Tuition assistance
- Career development opportunities
- Career ladders and parallel path progression
- Succession planning programs.

Separating Employees, including:
- Retirement processes
- Discharge and dismissal processes
- Terminal benefits processing (e.g., COBRA)
- Outplacement services
- Unemployment compensation
- Exit interviews.

Maintaining Employees

A great many Human Resources activities are intended to support employees by addressing the needs that arise relative to employment. Included in those activities are: compensation and benefits administration, personnel policies and procedures, disciplinary processes and other corrective processes, grievance procedures, personnel record keeping, administration of worker's compensation and disability programs, employee assistance programs, labor relations activities, security and parking, numerous forms of employee communication, and in general any other service that may be provided for the purpose of maintaining employees as effective producers.

Retaining Employees

There can of course be significant overlap between *retaining* employees and *maintaining* employees. For example, consider compensation and benefits. If compensation is not perceived as fair for the particular position or equitable when compared with other positions or with community standards, compensation will then do little to keep employees in the organization. Likewise, if benefits are clearly less than other employers are providing, then benefits will have little or no effect in retaining employees. The importance of compensation and benefits in retaining employees is embodied in the need to keep these competitive so that valued employees will be encouraged to remain.

Immediate monetary compensation, that is, pay and benefits, are not all it takes to keep good employees. Numerous other functions, activities, or perquisites intended to help retain employees often include: retirement plans, performance appraisal and performance management programs, award and recognition programs, training and development opportunities, career development and succession planning programs, employee assistance programs (important in both maintaining and retaining employees), tuition assistance programs, child care assistance, physical safety and security, and reasonable parking facilities.

Separating Employees

This category comprises all activities involved in separating employees from the organization, regardless of the reasons for separation. All kinds of separations involve paperwork and filing. Discharge for cause will require that disciplinary processes be carried out, as well as perhaps subsequent activities involving external agencies; layoffs will usually involve activities related to unemployment compensation, and possibly outplacement activities; retirements may involve counseling and administrative work related to a pension plan (and perhaps retirement celebrations to arrange); most voluntary separations will require exit interviews; and most separations will likely require activities associated with the end (or possible continuation of) certain benefits.

THE MANAGER'S INVOLVEMENT WITH HUMAN RESOURCES

The department manager can expect to come into regular contact with Human Resources people and processes at various times and for a variety of activities.

In general the department manager can expect:

- Frequent contact and considerable involvement in activities involving employment, employee relations, and labor relations (if unions are involved), and perhaps periods of active involvement with training and development
- Some involvement in activities involving compensation, benefits, safety, employee health, and payroll
- Little or no involvement in security, parking, child care, risk management, and a number of other HR concerns (except of course as an individual employee using some of these services).

It is in the department manager's best interests to learn how to do a better, more thorough job as a manager by using the services of Human Resources to the fullest extent possible.

The background, education, and experience of most department managers tends to reside in their technical or professional specialties. Some will also have general business knowledge, but most will not be familiar with Human Resources processes and requirements. Nevertheless, a certain amount of HR knowledge and involvement with HR is necessary if the manager is to manage the department's employees effectively.

Employment

In this area of active management contact with HR, the department manager must remain involved in recruitment and employment processes as a normal part of managing. How intense this activity becomes for the individual manager will depend largely on the turnover rate in the department.

When the manager finds it necessary to acquire a new employee, the manager's initial step, after creating or updating a job description (and before Human Resources comes into the picture), will often be securing approval of a personnel requisition from higher management. In some instances it may be possible for the manager to submit a personnel requisition directly to HR if it happens to be for a direct replacement for a departing employee; this depends on the practices of the organization. If the requisition is asking for an added employee, however, it usually requires thorough justification and subsequent approval by higher line management.

When Human Resources receives the personnel requisition it will be assigned to an employment recruiter, who will begin to identify an appropriate number of candidates. The department manager's next involvement is usually when HR supplies the manager with several applications or résumés of applicants who meet at least the stated minimum requirements of the job. The manager then reviews these and advises the HR recruiter which ones should be called for interviews.

The Human Resources recruiter will perform screening interviews and set up interviews with appropriate candidates with the department manager. Following interview (see Chapter 7, How to Conduct a Legal—but Effective—Selection Interview, for details), the manager conveys a choice to the recruiter and comes to agreement with the recruiter on starting pay, other details of a formal job offer, and the preferred starting date for the new employee.

For a variety of reasons, formal offers of employment originate only from Human Resources. An offer is ordinarily made contingent upon positive references and the applicant passing a pre-employment physical examination. Once an applicant has been completely cleared and begins work, it falls to the department manager to ensure that the new employee is oriented to the department and properly started on the job in all other respects.

Benefits

The department manager will have no active role in administering employee benefits. However, because employees generally view the department manager as their primary source of information about the organization as well as about the job, the manager can expect to regularly receive questions about benefits from employees. Accordingly, the manager needs to have some level of familiarity with the more commonly accessed benefits such as paid time off (vacation, sick leave, holidays, etc.).

There are actually two levels of knowledge about benefits that will stand the manager in good stead: (1) knowing the general benefits structure, and (2) for more complex questions—concerning, for example, worker's compensation or short-term disability—knowing the appropriate person in HR to whom the employee should be referred.

Compensation

The department manager needs to be familiar with the compensation structure as it affects the pay of all the department's employees—what the scales are, what they mean, where the employees are relative to the scales, and where each employee stands regarding compensation when compared with others who are similarly situated (similar work, similar length of employment, etc.). The manager should have sufficient knowledge of the compensation structure to be able to recognize when inequities have crept into the department's pay rates and to question these inequities with Human Resources.

The department manager and the individual employee on the job are the primary repositories of knowledge of how an individual job is performed, so the manager must be able to apply this knowledge in creating and maintaining job descriptions. An accurate, up-to-date job description is a necessity for determining the pay grade and range for any particular job; this essential part of compensation administration falls largely on the manager. Human Resources ordinarily participates in writing and updating job descriptions but cannot create quality job descriptions without departmental input; the best information about how a job is performed resides with the person who does the job and the manager who directs the individual in doing that job.

Employee Relations

Each time a problem concerning or involving an employee arises, there is the potential for the department manager's involvement with Human Resources. This involvement can come about because of: internal complaints made by or about employees and others, whether informal or formal (e.g., grievances); complaints lodged externally with agencies such as the state human rights division or the Equal Employment Opportunity Commission or originating as lawsuits; disciplinary actions originating with the department manager; and various other sources of involvement.

One regularly recurring employee-related activity that requires the manager's direct collaboration with Human Resources is performance appraisal. Human Resources ordinarily administers the appraisal system, keeps the system up to date, provides training in the system's use, and follows up on appraisal completion. The manager's role is to perform the appraisals of direct reporting employees according to the guidelines established by HR and in accordance with established timetables.

Personnel Records

Human Resources of course maintains the personnel records, but the department manager has certain regular areas of contact with personnel records. Much of what gets filed comes to HR from the department manager; foremost among these items are performance appraisals and disciplinary actions. In addition, the manager occasionally needs to review something in the personnel record of a present employee or to review the work record and qualifications of an employee who is seeking to transfer into the department.

HUMAN RESOURCES AND THE ORGANIZATION

It is no secret that in many work organizations, health care providers being no exception, there is a degree of strain, at times even some animosity, between Human Resources and the management of the line departments. Often these differences simply slow down or mildly frustrate the normal conduct of business. Occasionally, however, the differences lead to out-and-out antagonism that can significantly interfere with the efficient conduct of business.

"Line managers and staff human resource professionals spend a great deal of time talking *at* each other and often *past* each other and privately questioning each other's views about what goals and values are important."[1] Why are there sometimes such differences between HR and department management? Perhaps an examination of the differences between line management and Human Resources may help generate an understanding of why there is sometimes a credibility gap between the two.

Department Managers and Human Resources Practitioners Compared

Much of the tension between line management and human resources practitioners can be attributed to their different educational backgrounds and general work orientation.

Background and Qualifications

Backgrounds of HR practitioners are generally varied. Relatively few, but an increasing number over the past decade or two, have been educationally prepared specifically for Human Resources. A number of different academic backgrounds may be found in Human Resources—psychology, social psychology, sociology, organizational behavior, industrial relations, education, and others. HR practitioners are far less likely to be educated in specific technical or medical fields than are line department managers.

Department managers tend to be prepared in specific technical or professional occupations, invariably the functions they manage. On average the HR practitioner's education has been liberal and non-specifically focused. If it can be called "scientific" at all, we would have to refer to it as "soft" science, while the line manager's education tends to have been narrowly and specifically focused within what can often be referred to as "hard" science. At times the difference in background can be described as being as fundamental as the difference between concept and fact or between theory and practice.

Staff Managed

Line managers frequently have to manage a variety of people who bring a mix of values onto the job. Some of these people will need close, nearly constant supervision, while some are capable of working independently. The manager's group may also include an extremely broad mix of skills and educational backgrounds; consider, for example, the nurse manager who may supervise a group including masters-prepared nurse practitioners, registered nurses, licensed practical nurses, nursing assistants, and clerical personnel.

In Human Resources, on the other hand, we ordinarily find a group that is, first, considerably smaller than most line departments, and second, a relatively cohesive group composed of people who share similar values and a common outlook.

Management Style and Approach

The manager of a line department will ordinarily tend to manage with a downward orientation, with much management accomplished on a one-to-one basis. The downward orientation clearly marks the manager most of the time as "above" the workers in the overall scheme of operation. The manager may sometimes have to perform as a practitioner but, depending on department size and workload, in many instances this will be a relatively minor part of the role.

In Human Resources, with the exception of clerical support staff, the employees—the HR practitioners—are more likely to view themselves as colleagues on a comparable level with each other rather than as part of a hierarchical structure. In essentially all health care settings except the largest (e.g., health systems, teaching hospitals), the chief HR officer is likely to have his or her own practitioner duties as well and thus be regarded by the others much of the time as an organizational equal.

Expectations

The expectations placed on line management are relatively clear and usually easy to define. Line management is expected to do the assigned job in a manner that ensures consistency of quality and output while adhering to the policies of the organization and remaining faithful to the mission, vision, and goals of the organization.

The expectations of Human Resources may not be nearly as clear or recognizable as those placed on the line departments. Whether it is perceived that HR is expected to control, retain the status quo, avoid "making waves," or innovate will influence whether the line departments regard HR with apprehension, indifference, contempt, or caution. As long as the expectations of HR and the line departments differ noticeably from each other, there is likely to be some degree of tension between the functions.

Orientation and Training

In regard to matching the appropriate person to each task to be done, line management tends toward the belief that *selection* is the most important factor—that what is most important in getting a job done is selecting the right person to do it. Human Resources practitioners, on the other hand, tend to believe that *development* is the most important factor, i.e., that with proper development, any of several people can usually get the job done. This sometimes leads to sharp differences between line management and HR in the area of recruiting: Human Resources may have supplied several candidates who could do the job as expected if properly developed, but none is precisely the "right" person to the manager because the manager, knowingly or otherwise, is holding out for the "ideal" fit between candidate and position.

Participation

Line management frequently exhibits a tendency to believe that employee participation is a "management theory" notion that complicates matters, slows things down, and generally fails to contribute. HR practitioners, however, usually believe that participation, if properly pursued, can generate improved organizational performance and increased employee satisfaction.

Employee Empowerment

Line management, whose highest priority is getting the work done—in health care, taking care of patients—is often hesitant to delegate important tasks, frequently taking a "the-buck-stops-here" approach to everything perceived to be the manager's responsibility. Human Resources, however, whose highest priority is to *support* the performance of the work, will often advocate employee empowerment as a vehicle for employee growth and development in the belief that in order to grow, people need the freedom to fail.

Control

Line managers frequently act in accordance with the belief that exercising control is protective of the department's staff and enhances the organization's ability to deliver. The Human Resources view, however, is that the controlling manager stifles creativity, discourages employee participation, and impedes employee growth and development.

Staff Performance

Line management, especially in departments having a considerable mix of staff skills, qualifications, and educational levels, will ordinarily have to deal with varying levels of performance, at times necessitating counseling, criticism, disciplinary action, and even termination. Such "people problems" can consume a considerable portion of the line manager's time. The Human Resources manager usually deals with professional and a few support personnel of comparable skills, making the people problems fewer and corrective actions far less necessary.

Reward Assumptions

Line management tends to believe that compensation is the most effective means of influencing performance. Human Resources practitioners tend to place organizational culture, supportive management, employee participation, and development opportunity above monetary compensation in creating employee motivation over the long run.

Regarding Change

The line management belief seems to be that effective change occurs slowly, over time, and that true organizational change is always slow and incremental. The HR view is generally that genuine organizational change is achievable and can occur in the short term if it is driven and supported by top management.

Outlook

The line management orientation ordinarily sees success or failure occurring in the short run, while the typical HR view usually involves a longer-term perspective.

What Results in Practice

To summarize the apparent differences between line management and Human Resources:

- Line management believes that Human Resources impedes progress by frequently obstructing what the department manager wants or needs to do, commonly citing laws saying why something cannot be done.
- Human Resources feels that department managers regularly try to end-run laws and policies and generally insist on doing things that could cause legal trouble for the organization.

What Can Be Done

Many rank-and-file employees, along with some department managers, do not trust Human Resources, to the extent that some employees will never go to Human Resources with their needs because they feel that doing so will endanger their employment. As a result, these employees never take advantage of the HR processes that are available to them. Also, many employees apparently do not see HR as a resource available to them, but rather view it as a function that relates primarily with their managers and thus serves mainly the corporate hierarchy.

Department management and Human Resources can both help their mutual situation by giving each other the benefit of the doubt concerning their motives—that HR's mission in life is not to obstruct and frustrate department management, and that department management is not pouring its energies into finding ways around Human Resources. Rather, each should try to use every instance of disagreement as an opportunity to learn where the other is coming from.

A top priority of Human Resources is—or decidedly should be— communicating how HR can be an important resource for all employees, rank-and-file as well as managers. If Human Resources is *not* communicating this critical information, department management and administration should takes steps to see that this *does* occur (see Chapter 18, Keeping Human Resources on Its Toes). The Human Resources department should never forget—and should never be allowed to forget—what it is there for: to represent employees and advocate for them, to ensure that management is aware of what the employees need to keep them motivated and performing, and to propose and champion those programs and services that appear to be most needed.

Discussion Points

1. Outline a long-term approach for narrowing any credibility gap that might exist between an organization's Human Resources department and its department managers.
2. Advance an argument either for or against having the employee health and safety function reporting within the Human Resources division.
3. Describe the activity of "risk management" and state why you believe it is or is not essential in today's health care organization.

4. Explain why it is common practice to outsource the administration of the organization's Employee Assistance Program (EAP).
5. List several elements of a hypothetical "organizational development" program, and explain how and why such a program differs from "management development."
6. Discuss why it is preferable for the department manager to respond directly to the majority of employees' HR-related questions, rather than simply telling them to "go ask Human Resources."
7. Describe "screening interviews" and explain where and why they are ordinarily conducted.
8. Provide several reasons why the department manager should be familiar with the organization's compensation scales, even though the manager is not expected to make specific salary quotations to prospective employees.
9. List three or four differing academic backgrounds that might be found among Human Resources practitioners, and state the advantages or disadvantages of each in equipping an individual to provide HR services.
10. Describe what "outplacement services" consist of, and explain why such services are almost always provided by an external vendor.

NOTES

[1]Barry D. Leskin, "Two Different Worlds," *Personnel Administrator,* Vol. 31, No. 12, December 1986, p. 58.

The Manager-Employee Relationship

This chapter—

- Reviews the heterogeneous composition typical of groups found in the majority of health care organization departments
- Promotes the value and importance of employee participation and input
- Compares and contrasts production-centered management and people-centered management, and recognizes that most health care activities require people-centered management
- Stresses the importance of the department manager remaining visible and available to the staff
- Discusses the value of a true "open-door" policy
- Describes the manager's essential downward (toward the employees) orientation as opposed to an upward (toward higher management) orientation
- Conveys the importance of establishing and maintaining a solid one-to-one relationship with each employee in the department and the need to know each as a whole person to be an effective people-centered manager
- Introduces the department manager's key role in employee retention.

EVERY MANAGER IS A MANAGER OF HUMAN RESOURCES

Some managers, particularly those who hold to an old-fashioned (and inappropriately narrow) view of management, regard many em-

ployee-related concerns as something they might call "employee relations" rather than "management." Their concept of management is
entirely what we can refer to as production-centered, that is, concerned first, foremost, and always with getting the work done.

In organizations where Human Resources practitioners are used to
the maximum possible extent, some managers have come to rely so
heavily on Human Resources that by default they have conferred upon
HR the primary responsibility for addressing all people-related issues. However, regardless of the HR department's strength and relative position in the organization, day-to-day employee concerns and
everyday involvement in employee matters belong largely to department management.

This is not to say that Human Resources should not always be available for advice and assistance; this, after all, is much of the HR role.
However, there are any number of issues involving employees that
should not be allowed to automatically default to Human Resources.
Everyday people-related tasks are simply part of the manager's job.

HR does not in any way "manage" the people who do the work. In
providing the organization's "people systems," literally the processes
and procedures for serving all employees, HR simply provides the
framework within which relations with employee are conducted.

The Heterogeneous Work Group

Workers in health care organizations represent an extremely broad
range of educational backgrounds and levels of sophistication. Within
the same group of direct-reporting employees, a manager may have:

- Employees who require regular or even constant supervision
- Employees who are self-determining much of the time and need
  only the most general direction.

Consider some examples in many hospital organizations:

- In *food service*, there is often a mix of employees ranging from
  entry-level, on-the-job-trained food-service aides to master's degree therapeutic dietitians. Here a manager may be responsible
  for several levels of staff that exhibit their own different needs.
- In *diagnostic imaging* (radiology), employees may range from entry-level clerks and transporters to highly skilled special-proce-

dures technologists and even physicians who do not report directly to the manager. The manager in this venue may be responsible for as many levels of staff as the food service manager, while also relating to physicians who can be either medical staff members or employees of the organization.

- In *patient billing* and *housekeeping*, a single manager may be responsible for a number of personnel who are all at the same level of education and sophistication.
- In even a modest size *nursing unit*, the nurse manager may have several levels of staff: nursing assistants and unit clerks, licensed practical nurses (LPNs), registered nurses (RNs), and perhaps nurse clinicians.

In addition to multiple levels of education and sophistication, the heterogeneous work group can present the manager with another potentially troublesome condition—differences among employees regarding work ethic. Significant differences sometimes appear in work ethic between, for instance, newer employees and those who are more established, or older (in age) members of the group and younger workers. Although peoples' attitudes toward work and employment have on average shifted over the course of several generations, all problems related to work ethic are not assignable to younger, newer workers.

Variations in work ethic suggest that within the same group the manager may have some employees who would never willingly miss a day's work and never intentionally shirk a responsibility, and some employees who think nothing of missing work on a whim and allowing responsibilities to go unfulfilled. In addition to working to bring the best out of each employee, the department manager must serve as an example of a continually positive work ethic.

Employee Participation and Input

An anonymous individual once claimed that "When all is said and done there's much more said than done." In few circumstances does this hold truer than in employee participation. From time to time virtually all managers claim that they believe in employee participation and remain open to employee input. However, for the most part their behavior contradicts their words. They are saying what they believe they ought to say because it is what the "experts" are saying about modern management, especially in the best-selling management books that come along periodically. Yet they are simply "speaking Management 101," saying what they believe they are expected to say while they continue to behave in the same old way.

Managers who speak of their belief in participation only to tolerate it just superficially in practice may believe themselves to be participative managers when in fact their style is consultative. The consultative manager—who may be honest, conscientious, and completely well intended—simply cannot let go of enough control to allow employees to participate to their full potential. To managers who behave in this fashion, any experience or process that involves sharing authority or control with employees smacks of abrogation of responsibility; it is perceived as weakness. Participation is stifled by the streak of authoritarianism remaining in modern management.

Management has evolved for decades and will continue to evolve for decades to come. At the start of the twentieth century, management, for all practical purposes, was largely authoritarian in most settings: The boss was the boss, and the boss was to be obeyed. Period. The human relations movement in management, a twentieth century phenomenon, began to take hold in the 1930s, 1940s, and 1950s and has steadily expanded. Many who manage today have been educated specifically for management, but like those above them and others who have preceded them, they have acquired much of their management perspective from their working role models. It is not surprising to find residual authoritarianism in many who manage today; after all, their role models were at least partly authoritarian, as were *their* role models. This strain of authoritarianism in management is steadily weakening, but it is far from gone.

Concerning employee participation, the department manager should always make it clear to the employees that their ideas are valued and their input is not only welcome but needed. Even if one is to remain largely a consultative manager, reserving the right of final decision, it will still pay in the long run to solicit employee input, consider it carefully, and occasionally use employee ideas.

One fact of working life that is essential for the department manager to learn along the way is that when it comes to sources of knowledge about how to perform the work better, faster, or more economically, there is nobody who knows the inner workings of a job better than the person who does it day in and day out. The most successful managers are those who have learned how to tap this source of knowledge.

THE PEOPLE-FOCUSED MANAGER

Depending on the particular work environment and the kinds of work performed, a manager will tend toward being either production-centered or people-centered. In a production-centered situation (manufacturing, for example), the work is ordinarily highly repetitive, many units of output are similar, output can be scheduled with some accuracy, and jobs can be rigidly defined in great detail. In a production-centered situation, the people are ordinarily assigned to certain work stations and themselves have little control other than keeping up with what is expected of them. Picture, if you will, an assembly line: It is the speed of the line that determines rate of output, and if one particular employee does not keep pace, another is placed at that work station. In the production-centered situation, the manager's priority concerns are usually keeping supplies and services entering the process and thus keeping the output flowing. In the production-centered situation, the processes control the people, and the production-centered manager's primary focus is on output.

In the people-centered situation, it is not the pace at which the work arrives or the manner of supplying the processes that keeps the work flowing; rather, it is the willingness of the people to work that maintains output. In a people-centered situation, the work is irregular and varied, hardly any two units of output are identical, it is not possible to schedule output with true accuracy, and jobs defy rigid definition because demands on the workers can vary so broadly. In the people-centered situation, the people control the processes, and the people-centered manager's primary focus is on people—the producers.

In the health care organization most situations require people-centered management. People control the processes, and thus people must be the primary focus of the health care manager. The following few sections present some of the principal requirements of an effective people-centered manager—that is, an effective manager of health care workers.

Exhibit 5-1 compares and contrasts production-centered management and people-centered management in several dimensions. Based on the characteristics encountered in the majority of health care de-

Exhibit 5-1   Production-Centered Management versus People-Centered Management

	Production-Centered	People-Centered
Nature of the work	Repetitive	Variable
Nature of the output	Homogeneous	Heterogeneous
Pace controlled by	Process	People
Character of labor	More manual	More intellectual
Manager's primary focus	Process	People
Arrival of work	More predictable	Less predictable
Completion of work	Predictable intervals	Irregular intervals

livery settings, it is evident that most circumstances encountered in health care call for people-centered management.

Visibility and Availability

The health care department manager needs to be generally visible to employees and *perceived* as available as well as being actually available. The matter of perception is stressed because much of a manager's state of being visible and available is psychological as far as employees are concerned. Although it may never be articulated by employees, there is a level of comfort in seeing the manager around the department and knowing that this manager can be accessed should the need arise. Many of the employees may be able to work independently for prolonged stretches and may even prefer to do so, but on those occasions when the manager's judgment or expertise is required, they should at least know how to reach the manager in a reasonably short time. Also, and for what we hope will be a relatively few employees, the manager's presence in and around the work group will tend to limit certain kinds of inappropriate behavior.

Consider the case of the manager who looked forward to moving from her small, glass-encased cubicle in the corner of the department to new and larger quarters some distance away from her staff. Formerly all employees in the department could see whether the manager was available, but after the move it was impossible to know her availability without leaving the department and traveling some 300 feet of corridor. Within weeks following the move, complaints about the manager had noticeably increased—"Now she's hard to find when we need her"; "She pays more attention to higher management than to us"; "She no longer cares about us and our needs—look how she couldn't wait to get away from us." Over the weeks and months that followed, staff absenteeism and tardiness increased, productivity decreased, and interpersonal problems between and among staff members increased.

"Absentee management" may be appropriate in some retail business situations, but it is never appropriate in managing a department of people in an organizational situation.

A manager can create communication problems by not being reasonably accessible. When employees are forced to either wait to get answers or to take chances and act independently, time and perhaps material resources are wasted through delay and error. This can be especially troublesome in emergencies when time must be devoted to tracking down the missing manager.

The department manager should be perceived as the employees' direct line of communication with other organizational elements, especially with higher management. The manager who is not readily visible or available or who seems dedicated primarily to activities occurring away from the department (meetings, committee, conferences, etc.) can be perceived by the employees as uninterested, uncaring, perhaps even cold and distant but certainly indifferent and impersonal. To many members of the work group, the department manager is representative of the organization itself: This manager is the one member of management these employees know best and perhaps the *only* member of management with whom they have a speaking relationship. If the employees perceive the manager as cold, uncaring, and impersonal, so too are they likely to perceive the entire organization.

Also, the first-line manager is in most instances a worker as well as a manager, if not regularly at least from time to time, and is thus an additional resource to the department. When the manager is unavailable, a productive resource is unavailable.

A Genuine Open Door

Hardly a manager exists who has not taken occasion to say, "My door is always open," regardless of that person's individual style. Many espouse it, but few are able to practice a true open-door policy. Managers are usually busy people, especially in these days of shrinking managerial hierarchies and expanding responsibilities. There are problems to wrestle with, meetings to attend, telephone calls to take and make, and generally many time-consuming activities that render it impossible for the manager to sit behind a desk inside a physically open door just waiting for employees to drop in.

Some managers cannot be readily accessed at the will of the employee because they are genuinely too busy. Some cannot be accessed because even though the manager has said, "My door is always open," the manager's *attitude* says, "The door may stand open, but I dislike interruptions and you had best not enter without an appointment."

Even the manager who is generally visible and available to employees most of the time can discourage contact by projecting an attitude that discourages employees from approaching.

An honest open door is easier to maintain for the first-line manager than for higher management. A first-line manager can usually directly address many problems and issues that are brought in via the open door. Higher levels of management, however, need to exert greater care in addressing issues brought directly by rank-and-file employees because of an espoused open-door policy. Whatever higher management does must not subvert the authority of an employee's immediate manager, so the higher manager's response must often be to refer the matter down to the first-line supervisor or other source of assistance (e.g., Human Resources).

It is best to make it as easy as possible for the department's employees to access their manager. As a first-line manager, remain appropriately visible and available and strive to offer a reasonably accessible open door. Observe the open door whenever you are able to do so, and when not readily available make it possible for employees to get specific appointments for you to meet with them.

Show, Don't Tell

A similar inconsistency between what a manager says and what that manager actually does occurs with the manager who espouses a belief in participative management. The very first instance in which the manager fails to—or is unable to—allow employee participation, again there is immediately perceived inconsistency between the manager's words and the manager's actions.

Today's manager is subject to the very nearly constant temptation to say "the right things," to repeat those phrases that are well-intended to convey the impression that employees always stand high among the manager's concerns. These proper statements represent people-centered management right out of the textbooks. However, no matter how well-intentioned a manager may be, it is not always possible to completely live up to what might be said, even though it may be spoken with utmost sincerity, so such statements create inconsistencies that most employees eventually recognize. When these inconsistencies between what one says and what one does become evident, the contradictory perceptions created lead some employees to see only that the leader has claimed one guiding belief but has acted contrary to that belief. When this occurs, the leader's credibility suffers.

Whether any particular individual employee's perception of the manager's behavior is correct, partly correct, or not at all correct, is irrelevant. What is relevant is the perception. If an employee perceives the leader as untruthful for saying one thing and acting contrary to it, to that employee the perception represents the truth.

It rarely pays for a manager to tell employees what kind of leader he or she is; this invariably leads to negative perceptions at the first sign of contrary behavior. Do not attempt to verbalize your supposed "leadership style" to employees; rather, let them infer your style of leadership from your behavior on the job. In brief, do not tell them what kind of leader you are—show them.

The Essential Downward Orientation

Strongly related to visibility and availability is the perception of whether the department manager is oriented upward or downward in the organizational structure. There is a strong natural attraction for the individual manager to be upwardly oriented, that is, "facing upward" much of the time in the direction of the manager's organizational superiors. This is natural to a considerable extent because it is the hierarchy above the manager—the manager's manager and other organizational superiors—that controls much of what the individual manager desires. It is from above that the department manager receives praise and reward and secures a certain amount of organizational status and promotional visibility, and it is often this association with the hierarchy from which the manager receives an enhanced feeling of importance and self-worth.

The forces encouraging a manager to face upward can be strong. Often not nearly as strong are pressures to face downward toward the immediate work group and its needs. However, downward is the direction in which the department manager must look for the primary reasons for the existence of his or her management position. The manager is the leader of this group of people who do the hands-on work and depend on this leader for guidance. So the manager's primary orientation should be downward, toward his or her own department and employees and the clients they serve. The manager is primarily the leader of the department's employees and is only secondarily a member of the greater hierarchy called "management."

The manager who is career-minded, seeking to advance within the organization, is often inclined to seek the visibility obtained by facing upward. It is of course better for all concerned in the long run if the department manager remains solidly oriented downward, displaying an obvious interest in accomplishing the work of the department. It is the managers who face downward, truly leading the employees, who turn out the best work and gain the most valuable experience for themselves. Yet we can hardly blame some for resenting the way the organizational system seems to work when a manager who rightly faces downward, paying attention to "minding the store," sees another who has achieved higher visibility by facing upward—some might describe the posture as "kissing up"—promoted to the next level of management. Simple visibility coupled with one's ability to "talk a good job" has led to the promotion of many managers of limited capability. However, truly effective upper management is more likely to promote based on operating results rather than on superficial indicators.

As with other elements of leadership style, employees will readily perceive whether their manager faces upward or downward. The manager who is clearly perceived as upward-facing is likely to be seen as separate from the group, insulated from the employees by virtue of being "management." The appropriately downward-facing manager is more readily acceptable to the employees as "one of our own," a full-fledged team member for whom they will willingly produce.

ESSENTIAL INDIVIDUAL RELATIONSHIPS

It is essential that the department manager cultivate and conscientiously maintain a one-to-one relationship with each employee. This must be done through conscious effort; an effective communicating relationship will not happen automatically. Establishing and maintaining such a relationship with each employee should be a key concern of the department manager, at times seeming to receive even higher priority treatment than departmental productivity. Productivity is of course always a priority concern, so it follows that the maintenance of the department's productive capacity should rate a high priority—and in an activity as labor-intensive as health care, a department's productive capacity resides in its people.

One of the most effective means of maintaining a labor-intensive department's productive capacity is to ensure that each employee is given reason to feel like a full-fledged contributing member of a team. This calls for a deliberately forged and maintained relationship between the manager and each employee, excluding none (but perhaps those who will occasionally exclude themselves).

Most department managers are busy people with sometimes more demands coming at them than can reasonably be met on any given work day. This being so, some managers exhibit a tendency to ignore those employees who simply go along day after day doing their jobs in reasonably acceptable fashion, never acting out and never causing trouble. Troublesome employees, although relatively few in number, often consume inordinate amounts of the manager's time.

Consider who in a work group gets noticed and who does not. The relatively few employees who may perform outstandingly are usually noticed, and although they do not necessarily consume much of the manager's time, they surely get the manager's attention. The troublesome employees—those who consistently make mistakes and exhibit performance problems as well as those who violate work rules or policies—are noticed *and* they consume time. The vast majority between the outstanding performers and the troublesome employees are frequently not noticed and thus get little or none of the manager's time and attention. We can perhaps correctly state that the age-old Pareto Principle—the so-called "80/20 rule"—applies to this dimension of manager-employee relationships in that 20 percent or fewer of employees consume 80 percent or more of the manager's time. That 80 percent of employees in the middle go along day after day doing acceptable work, rarely outstanding but always acceptable, and never causing problems, so the "quiet ones" are for all practical purposes ignored.

However, even the "quiet ones" require the manager's attention if they are to remain acceptable producers and non-troublesome employees. Relationships with them need to be maintained or often they will deteriorate on their own.

Other than addressing task-related matters, some managers meet face-to-face with individual employees on just two kinds of occasions:

performance appraisal meetings, which usually occur only once per year; and when it becomes necessary to address a problem via counseling, disciplinary action, or other corrective processes. To one whose manager usually meets face-to-face with employees under these two sets of circumstances, hearing the invitation to "Come into my office" can raise considerable apprehension.

It is necessary to meet periodically with each employee even when there is no pressing business reason to do so. Some conversation about the job, some talk about the organization and its future and the department's role, and especially the opportunity for the employee to ask questions and air any perceived problems or complaints can all be instrumental in helping maintain a relationship with the individual. Even a few occasional minutes of simply social conversation, totally unrelated to work, can help nurture the one-to-one relationship.

We are of course suggesting that it is important to come to know each employee as a whole person, not just as a producer of output. Doing so not only ensures continued steady performance from the employee, but it provides additional advantages for the manager as well. By knowing each employee fairly well, the manager will acquire knowledge other than that normally associated with individual capabilities; the manager will learn who needs more guidance or assistance at times than others, who is sufficiently motivated to take on additional tasks or learn new things, who might seem to be the better prospects for promotion, and so on.

Regular communication with employees is a necessity for one who would become an effective employee-centered manager. This means communication in a variety of settings and personnel combinations: regular staff meetings that include the entire department; meetings of project teams, work-improvement teams, and various *ad hoc* groups; formal or semi-formal one-on-one meetings such as appraisal interviews and counseling and disciplinary sessions; and regular—preferably frequent—informal one-to-one conversations.

Also, to combine one's visibility and availability with frequent informal communication with employees, it can be extremely beneficial to simply get out into the department and talk with the employees in their own work setting. "Management by wandering around" remains an extremely effective employee relations practice.

We hear much about the need for teamwork in the effective delivery of health care as well as in various other endeavors. However, one does not forge a departmental team without also being attentive to the needs of individual employees. It is essential that the department manager strive to create a team environment in which each individual can be encouraged to feel an important element of the whole.

People who feel they are "on the inside," that they are an included, knowledgeable, and appreciated part of the team, will be more satisfied and productive than if they feel they have been excluded or otherwise "left outside." The manager's treatment of and relationship with each employee are the most important factors in determining whether an individual feels included or excluded.

THE COST OF IGNORED EMPLOYEES

Some managers have adopted an attitude regarding employees that suggests, "If this one doesn't work out, no problem—I can always hire another." Directly associated with such an attitude are costs that the manager may not be able to see immediately. Employees who are ignored or taken for granted contribute to turnover, and turnover has many costs associated with it, a few of them obvious but many of them indirect.

Although we may be hard put to measure some of these indirect costs with any accuracy, the following dimensions of turnover contribute to the overall cost of doing business:

- The diminishing efficiency of the individual who is preparing to leave
- The costs of separating the departing employee (exit interviews, severance pay if applicable, unemployment compensation if applicable, general out-processing, etc.)
- The value of the output lost while a position is vacant
- The inefficiency of a replacement employee while that person is getting up to speed
- Orientation and training, extra initial supervision, personally related equipment and supplies (identification badge, employee handbook, etc.)
- Human Resources department processing costs, including all related forms and paperwork
- Recruiting costs (recruitment literature, job fairs, recruiting trips, etc.)
- Processing costs (pre-employment physical examination, etc.)

- Travel and relocation expenses, if any (ordinarily for higher-level positions only)
- Agency fees or finders' fees
- General overhead associated with all these activities.

The cost of employee turnover is sometimes easy to overlook because so much of it is hidden. Turnover is disruptive as well as costly, and much of it is driven by how individuals feel about their employment and how they are treated. It therefore follows that employees are more likely to remain in their jobs if they:

- Feel valued as individuals and as producers
- Feel they are accepted as part of a group
- Find an acceptable amount of challenge and interest in the work
- See the opportunity for growth and advancement.

Generous benefits and employee-friendly programs will go only so far in retaining employees. One of the strongest influences in determining whether a particular employee remains or departs is the relationship that employee has with the department manager.

The individual feeling valued, being accepted, and finding challenge and interest in the work are entirely controllable by the manager. Depending on certain organizational policies, the manager may also have some influence on an employee's opportunity for growth and advancement. In the labor market within which health care has been operating for some time, top performers, especially professional and technical employees, rarely have much trouble finding new employment when they want it. For some occupations, in fact, other organizations are ready and willing to recruit your best people away from you.

Two aspects of the relationships the manager has with employees are critical in determining whether they wish to remain or depart: how they are treated and how they are used. How they are treated as individuals can be assumed to be of essentially equal importance to all employees; generally, fair and respectful treatment is positive for all employees, while the opposite makes negative impressions on all employees. How employees are used seems to vary in its effects according to the level of enthusiasm and motivation of the individual. That is, being challenged, having their ideas heard, being given responsibility, and having growth opportunity are of most importance to the better performers. And it is of course the better performers that the manager should be seeking to retain. Some depart along the way for reasons of career advancement, but it is far better to lose good performers this way than for them to depart prematurely out of dissatisfaction.

Individuals will not remain long in an organization if they feel unwelcome or excluded, or otherwise feel there is little opportunity for them. One of the most important factors in determining whether a valued producer will choose to remain or depart is that individual's relationship with his or her immediate supervisor—the department manager.

Discussion Points

1. Explain the concept that every manager is—or should be—a manager of "human resources."
2. Describe a health care organization department comprising a heterogeneous work group consisting of at least three differing levels of staff (differing in educational background and job responsibility).
3. Explain in detail what is meant by the statement: "Participation is stifled by the streak of authoritarianism remaining in modern management."
4. Provide two or three examples each of activities you believe could thrive under production-centered management or proceed most appropriately under people-centered management.
5. Identify the biggest problem usually associated with a manager's claim to the practice of an open-door policy.
6. Explain why it is necessary for the department manager to pay attention to the employees who steadily fulfill their responsibilities and cause no problems.
7. Comment on the statement: "This is a simple job we're filling, a no-brainer," the department manager said, "so just send me any warm body, and if this one doesn't work out we can always get someone else and we've lost nothing."
8. Explain why the department manager's visibility and availability to employees is considered important.

9. Explain how a department manager comes to know which employees require what kinds of attention at what times.
10. If "teamwork" is so critically important in today's health care organization, discuss why such strong emphasis is placed on the one-to-one relationship between the manager and each employee.

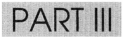

PART III

Obtaining Employees

CHAPTER 6

The Manager and the Recruiting Process

This chapter—

- Reviews the various steps in the recruiting process
- Describes the essential partnership between the department manager and Human Resources in recruiting employees
- Cautions the department manager about active involvement in checking references or answering references requests, introducing the concepts of defamation and negligent hiring
- Reviews the department manager's role in finding job candidates
- Addresses the advantages and disadvantages of promoting from within the organization
- Reviews some special recruiting concerns, such as recruiting during periods of labor shortage.

LEGAL CONCERNS IN RECRUITING

Many of the laws outlined in Chapter 3 exert considerable influence on the employment process. Especially pertinent are those having to do with equal employment opportunity (EEO), particularly Title VII of the Civil Rights Act of 1964.

Much of the legislation reviewed thus far is primarily the concern of the Human Resources Department; however, there are implications for the department manager throughout, and a great deal for the manager to be aware of in conducting interviews of prospective employees. (Interviewing is addressed in detail in Chapter 7, "How to Conduct a Legal—But Effective—Selection Interview.")

IN PARTNERSHIP WITH HUMAN RESOURCES

Obtaining employees is an area of activity in which the department manager and Human Resources usually work closely together. Although the process may vary somewhat from one organization to another, the following discussion is representative of a fairly standard recruiting relationship between Human Resources and the organization's departments.

Initially the department manager provides an approved personnel requisition to Human Resources. The requisition may call for a replacement for an employee who is resigning, retiring, or being discharged, or it may call for an employee to fill a position that did not previously exist. Depending on the nature of the requisition, the department manager will take a few necessary steps before HR receives the requisition:

- In the majority or organizations, if the request is for a new employee (that is, one who represents an addition to the department's work force), the department manager will be expected to go through a justification process to secure approval for an added position from higher management. This process may or may not involve input from Human Resources, but HR usually will be unable to recruit without higher management's approval.
- In some organizations, if the need is for a direct replacement, the department manager is empowered to initiate the requisition and submit it directly to Human Resources.
- In organizations that are undergoing reengineering or experiencing financial difficulties, higher management may choose to review positions that come open and determine whether they should be allowed to go unfilled. In this environment, higher management may reserve the right to review and approve of *all* requests for staff, even direct replacements.

Once a personnel requisition is approved, the department manager submits it to Human Resources. If the requisition is to replace a retiring employee or one who has been discharged, Human Resources will expect the requisition because HR will have been involved in processing the retirement or the discharge. If the requisition is for an employee to fill a newly created position, HR might not have received advance notification.

The next step involves the job description for the position in question. If the requisition is for a direct replacement that HR knew of in advance, HR will usually have pulled the appropriate job description, reviewed it, and asked the department manager to examine it for possible updating. If the requisition is for a newly created position, HR will expect to receive a new job description along with it or immediately following. It is usually the responsibility of the department manager to provide an accurate job description, either new or updated as appropriate. Often Human Resources will be able to assist in developing or updating a job description, but it should be obvious that most of the information necessary for doing so will reside in the line department and not in HR.

An accurate job description is essential in getting the recruiting process properly underway. Human Resources will need to have a grasp of the position's major duties for purposes of job posting (seeking internal applicants, if possible) and advertising (for external applicants). Also, as soon as people begin to apply and screening interviews are underway, HR will need the information from the job description to be able to describe the position accurately to applicants.

So at the time an approved personnel requisition is submitted, the department manager should have available, preferably incorporated in a comprehensive job description:

- An accurate, up-to-date description of job duties
- A checklist of the experience and qualifications to look for in the individuals to be interviewed.

In addition, the department manager should be prepared to:

- Consider appropriate internal as well as external candidates
- Interview the several apparent best prospects for the position in question
- Have applicants' references checked and academic credentials verified as necessary.

When a personnel requisition arrives in Human Resources, the initial consideration may be to determine whether the position is to be posted internally. Most organizations, especially large ones, operate job posting systems by which present employees may apply for open positions that represent transfer or promotional opportunities to them. In some places internal posting and external advertising will commence at the same time; frequently, however, the employer's posting system will provide a reasonable time—perhaps one work week, perhaps more—for internal candidates to apply before external candidates are considered. An exception may occasionally be encountered in the form of a position (usually a skilled technical or professional position) for which it is known there are no qualified employees available in-house; in this instance, the external search is started immediately upon receipt of the requisition.

Whether the job candidates are coming from inside or outside or both, is it the job of Human Resources to provide the department manager with a number of candidates who meet the stated minimum qualifications of the position. *How many* candidates should be provided for interview for any particular position will depend largely on the labor market at the time of recruiting. For some of the high-skill professions that are at times in short supply, it may be difficult to get even one or two viable candidates. For entry-level positions, Human Resources should be able to provide the department manager with five or six reasonable candidates without consuming too much time conducting screening interviews.

In hiring entry-level personnel, the department manager should be able to select one suitable employee from five or six candidates who meet the published minimum requirements of the position. However, HR and department management often differ in their view of how many candidates are reasonable. The occasional manager will go through five, ten, fifteen or more candidates, holding out for one who significantly exceeds the minimum requirements of the position. It would of course be a significant advantage for the manager to secure a superior employee who could arrive essentially fully trained and hit the ground running with minimal orientation. However, the "ideal" candidate rarely appears. Ordinarily the manager can do no better selecting one of five or six than wading through fifteen or twenty candidates, but every extra candidate means extra work and expense in the recruitment system.

In some organizations, instead of conducting many screening interviews Human Resources will begin by reviewing applications and sending the department manager a supply of applications of people who—at least on paper—possess the minimum qualifications of the job. The manager will review the applications and decide which candidates to interview. Some managers prefer to work in this manner, although it is slightly more work for them in that they are essentially doing their own initial screening as well as interviewing in depth.

HR's time spent finding and referring candidates, and the department manager's time spent interviewing, along with lost productivity and training and orientation activities, all represent costs of recruiting. These are indirect costs, but they are nevertheless real, so the extent to which department management and HR are able to cooperate in recruiting activities will have an effect on the efficiency and therefore the cost of the process.

Chapter 7 addresses the department manager's role in interviewing in considerable detail. At this point it is sufficient to offer a precaution that will be repeated in connection with concluding a selection interview: When meeting with a candidate, avoid discussing pay except in the most general terms, such as describing the pay range for the position, and do not attempt to explain benefits. Benefits information can get complicated, especially if the organization has a benefits structure that includes various choices, and HR is the only function prepared to address benefits options. Also—frequently a danger when a candidate interviews well and the manager is deciding this is the one to hire—do not presume to extend an offer of employment during the departmental interview. All offers ordinarily go through Human Resources, and formal offers must be extended conditionally, to be considered firm only upon successful reference checks and proper medical clearance via a pre-employment physical examination.

Another occasional point of contention between the department manager and Human Resources is the timeliness of getting the new employee on board once an offer is made and accepted. Some managers, for example, seem to feel that unless a candidate who accepts a formal offer has to work out a period of notice for another employer, that new person ought to be able to start work immediately.

Human Resources will ordinarily do everything reasonably possible to get each new employee on board quickly and efficiently, but even in these days of rapid communication it still requires a modest amount of time to check references. Also, HR is usually completely dependent on the organization's employee health service or employee health physician to provide time for a pre-employment physical exam.

At times Human Resources may be pressured by line management to short-cut the process by allowing the new hire to begin work immediately and take care of reference checking and the physical examination during the person's first two or three days of work. This practice is to be discouraged. If the person is already on the payroll when reference checks come back negative, it may not be possible to easily reverse the hiring decision. A contingent offer can be withdrawn before the person begins work, but once the person is hired the contingency is gone. If the individual fails the physical examination, removing the person from the job after officially starting presents some difficulties. Also, in many parts of the country, state codes prohibit a worker from starting employment in a health care facility without having passed a proper pre-employment physical examination.

REFERENCE CHECKING AND THE DEPARTMENT MANAGER

Assuming that the organization has a centralized activity like Human Resources, a department manager should not become personally involved in checking an applicant's references or answering reference requests. References are best checked, and reference information on past employees best given out, through a single, central point where the people doing so are familiar with all applicable laws, can check all pertinent applicants' references in a similar manner, and can respond to all reference information requests consistently.

Exchanging reference information is an area of occasional friction between Human Resources and department managers. On the surface, there would seem to be some rationale for allowing certain managers, for example, health professionals who manage health professionals, to exchange reference information with other organizations without HR intervention. To paraphrase a manager who insisted on personally requesting and dispensing reference information about high-tech employees: "It requires someone with my level of specialized knowledge to render judgments on an individual's capabilities." Ironically, however, this statement contains precisely the reason why such a manager should *not* become involved in exchanging reference information.

Judgments have no place in a response to a reference request. Reference responses should include no judgments, no opinions, nothing that is in any way subjective. Subjective statements can always be challenged, and seldom is it possible to substantiate a judgment in a way that renders it an absolute truth. The only information that is completely safe legally to give out in answering a reference check is information that can be verified in the personnel record, and then only if the information happens to be relevant to the request.

Reference requests are best answered by someone who has access to the personnel file, and preferably by someone who was not necessarily well acquainted with the employee. All reference requests should be answered impersonally and directly from the record. Legally, and therefore for all practical purposes, if something is not in the record, it never happened. Anything said in response to a reference request must be verifiable in the personnel file.

Many organizations have become so gun-shy about giving out reference information that they have adopted the practice of either not answering at all or limiting their answers to verification of job titles and dates of employment. Some organizations exhibit an obvious double standard concerning references: When checking references on potential new hires they try to obtain as much information from prior employers as possible, yet when responding to reference requests they limit their responses to as little as possible (dates and titles, and perhaps salary).

There are opposing sides to the legal dangers involved in giving and receiving reference information, one receiving far more attention than the other. The apparently more obvious risk—at least the side of the issue that seems to have made so many employers hesitant to dispense reference information—is the possibility of being charged with *defamation.* Many employers fear being sued by someone because of something said in a reference that allegedly caused the person to miss out on being hired by the requesting employer, so the responding employer limits answers to as little as possible.

The legal hazard on the other side of reference checking, apparently not nearly as high in the consciousness of employers as defamation, is the risk of charges of *negligent hiring.* Assume that an employer hires a new employee without checking references, but that employee had a record of serious misdeeds known to the former employer. If that employee then causes harm people or property while working for the organization that failed to check references, the organization is at risk for a negligent hiring charge. Also, there is a secondary danger to the person's past employer; if the past employer had relevant, documented knowledge of a serious problem (for example, assault or theft) and did not reveal that information upon request, there could be legal repercussions for this employer as well.

It is relatively common for someone to charge defamation, claiming that he or she did not get a desired position because of something said in a response to a reference request. A few such complaints become legal cases that can languish with advocacy agencies or in the courts for months or years. These are time-consuming and can get costly, and for department managers who chose to involve themselves in giving out reference information, the process can be extremely frustrating. This is perhaps the most compelling reason to leave all reference responses to Human Resources. Should a charge of defamation become a full-scale legal hassle, the frustration is then HR's, not the department manager's.

Legal actions involving negligent hiring are not nearly as common as those involving defamation, but the negligent hiring cases tend to be considerably more serious and decidedly more expensive.

Organizations are usually fairly safe in answering reference requests with documented truth from the personnel record, as long as what is said is pertinent in assessing the person for the job being sought and as long as the information is not conveyed with malicious intent.

Those who are charged with answering reference requests should not attempt to interpret the record but should simply respond directly with information from the record. For example, concerning attendance one might say "Absent 9 times and tardy 12 times in three months" but should never say "Frequently late or absent; can't be depended upon to be there when needed." As long as the former is in the record it cannot easily be disputed, but the latter is imprecise and includes judgment and opinion.

Even if there is no Human Resources department, which may well be the case in some small organizations, it is still best to address reference information centrally. This is best done by the person charged with maintaining the organization's personnel files (which themselves had best be centralized).

Regardless of precautions about dealing with reference information, there will always be tendencies among some managers to exchange such information among peers and colleagues. In most areas, local health care organizations tend to be well acquainted with each other. Managers likely attend conferences together and belong to the same professional organizations. As employees move about the community from employer to employer, it is natural for managers to speak with each other about employee capabilities. A manager who engages in such conversations—essentially trading reference information—should nevertheless observe the essential rule: Offer no judgments and convey nothing that cannot be verified in the personnel file.

Should you ever find yourself in the witness chair in federal court, under oath, and you are asked specific questions about a certain conversation with your friend and colleague, how will you answer? And how will your friend and colleague answer? Best to avoid the possibility altogether by leaving the giving and receiving of reference information to Human Resources.

THE MANAGER'S ROLE IN FINDING CANDIDATES

A constant concern of Human Resources is finding and retaining the kinds of talent the organization needs. This should also be a continuing concern for the department manager.

Advertising

Newspaper advertisements are not nearly as effective as some may believe, although they are probably the most readily visible means of finding candidates. The department manager and Human Resources often disagree regarding the frequency of advertising and the size of ads. Also, some managers tend to miss ad deadlines or to see them as unrealistic.

In most communities the Sunday newspaper is the best time to run employment advertising. The greatest number of employment ads run on Sunday, and the Sunday paper uses the greatest variety of ad sizes and types and usually includes special sections of interest (such as "Medical"). It is not uncommon for the newspaper's deadline for Sunday advertising, especially display ads, to be, for example, noon Thursday. Given the crush of business in both HR and the departments during almost any given week, it often becomes a rush to make the ad deadline—with managers sometimes unable to get an ad approved and accepted late Friday. Human Resources will frequently issue reminders of the ad deadline to managers whose departments have open personnel requisitions.

There are also special health care employment publications that are national, regional, and sometimes local, and there are nationally circulated professional journals that carry employment advertising. With these publications, however, especially with the professional journals, longer recruiting time is involved, largely because of publication schedules and thus longer lead times.

Some Human Resources employment recruiters have said that they obtain no more than one-third of new employees as a result of print advertising.

Networking

Technical, professional, and managerial positions are often filled through networking. Someone seeking a position makes personal contacts among friends, relatives, acquaintances, and former colleagues, and especially among people working within or in organizational proximity to one's field of interest. This spreads the word around that one is seeking a particular kind of position. By receiving networking referrals to other individuals from one's original and subsequent contacts, one can often meet with a series of individuals that he or she would not have been able to access directly. This series of contacts and referrals and more contacts constitutes the "network."

Employers also use networking to find people to fill specific positions. Recruiters actively network in search of potential job candidates at professional society meetings, conferences and conventions, and other gatherings of people who work in a particular field. Many department managers have made initial contact at such gatherings with people they later hired.

Networking also takes place at job fairs.

Job Fairs

Job fairs are gatherings of employers who are interested in gaining exposure for their organizations and promoting them as good places to work. A typical job fair is set up very much like the vendors' room at a convention, with each employer having a table and perhaps a display of information about the organization. An employer's table will be staffed by an employment recruiter from Human Resources and often a department manager or one or two employees of a particular specialty.

Job fairs can be sponsored by municipalities, business organizations, trade associations, Chambers of Commerce, colleges and universities, and other organizations. They are usually well publicized, and those who are invited to attend are reminded to bring a supply of current résumés. Schools that educate health care workers—for example, schools of nursing—often hold job fairs that are attended by its graduating seniors and local health care employers.

Recruiting Trips

A department manager may become involved in recruiting trips, usually in conjunction with Human Resources. These trips may involve going to certain conferences, conventions, colleges and universities, and other gatherings of whatever occupation the organization is seeking to recruit.

The department manager's participation in such trips can be essential in recruiting professional employees such as registered pharmacists, nurses, and physical therapists. On such a trip the HR recruiter provides information about the organization, and the department manager addresses questions asked professional-to-professional. Experience has shown that recruiting trips that involve a department manager or other professional from within the specific department being recruited for tend to be more successful than those made by an employment recruiter alone.

Search Firms

Search firms, frequently referred to as "headhunters," are often used to locate and acquire employees for certain hard-to-fill jobs, usually middle or upper management positions and professional positions that require skills that are in short supply on the labor market.

The department manager may have occasion to suggest the use of a search firm. However, Human Resources usually engages the search firm, most often only with administrative or executive concurrence. The costs associated with the use of search firms can run as high as 40 percent of a year's salary for the position filled. Given the fiscal climate within health care in recent years, many organizations use search firms only after other options have been exhausted.

PROMOTION FROM WITHIN

The top management of most organizations often espouses a philosophy of development and promotion from within the organization. Many health care organizations have written policies to this effect communicated to all employees. Such a policy recognizes that one of the job-related conditions important to many employees is the opportunity for promotion and growth.

Nonetheless, some department managers tend to look outside for their new employees most of the time. This practice frequently gives rise to conflict because employees hear one thing but see something different occurring in practice.

It is necessary to strike a balance between internal transfer and promotion and external recruiting. To a considerable extent it is healthy for an organization to fill many of its openings by people moving up, then recruiting to fill the entry-level positions vacated by those being promoted. However, filling all responsible positions through promotion from within can sometimes lead to a kind of organizational stagnation, as people who think and act in the manner of their organizational role models simply perpetuate that behavior. New blood is a necessity from time to time, and new blood comes from outside.

On the other hand, filling all of the better jobs from outside can demoralize the existing staff. One of the employment conditions important to many employees is the opportunity for promotion and growth within the organization. Employees will know whether this opportunity is or is not provided, and even many who might never take advantage of it are demoralized by its absence. The absence of the perceived opportunity for promotion and growth places a figurative ceiling on all employees' advancement potential.

Most Human Resources departments in health care operate a job posting system that keeps employees informed of promotion and transfer opportunities. It is appropriate in many instances to give employees a few days to bid on transfer or promotional possibilities before opening the jobs up to external applicants.

For non-technical, non-professional positions, especially those for which most expertise is developed through on-the-job training and experience, it is healthy for the organization to promote from within. This of course leaves entry-level openings that can then be filled from outside. This practice permits managers to fill positions of increasing responsibility with people who have proven themselves at entry level.

Perhaps some department managers tend to look externally much of the time because they are unsure that internal candidates, obviously untested at a higher level, can perform as required. However, that is a risk common to all placements, whether from inside or outside. Some highly experienced managers have hired some external candidates possessing marvelous qualifications who nevertheless turned out to be disasters. Internally, if one knew for certain that a particular person could handle the more responsible job, then the move might not represent a growth opportunity for the individual.

There is an additional reason why department managers are encouraged to look closely at potential internal candidates before looking to the outside. When a qualified internal candidate who falls into what is referred to as a "protected class" under equal employment opportunity (EEO) laws does not get a desired position which then goes to an external candidate, there is always the possiblity of charges of discrimination. Many HR practitioners have had to field formal complaints that boiled down to: "I didn't get the promotion because I'm _____." (Fill in the blank with the appropriate designation of race, creed, color, national origin, religion, gender, age, etc.) For this reason, and in support of development from within, department managers are encouraged to always look closely at qualified internal candidates before recruiting externally.

RECRUITING DURING PERIODS OF SHORTAGE

Recruiting becomes understandably more difficult during periods of low unemployment and when certain important skills are in short supply. When particular kinds of workers become hard to find, the labor market becomes a sellers' market, at least for those limited specialists who essentially have their choice of employers. Under such conditions several special approaches can be taken to attract new employees.

From time to time *internship programs* have proven to be an effective means of long-term recruiting for certain scarce professionals. For example, a hospital that provides an internship experience for one or two pharmacy students may find the students willing to return as employees after graduation. Someone who has had a positive internship experience is more likely to become an employee than a candidate to whom the organization is new and unfamiliar.

Moving *expenses* are often paid or partial *moving allowances* offered, usually for professional and managerial employees recruited from out of town. This is standard practice in recruiting top management personnel, and the scarcer certain professionals become the more likely the recruiting organizations are to offer such inducements.

Some organizations *assist spouses in finding employment* as part of the process of recruiting scarce professionals. Dual-career couples are becoming increasingly common, and some effort to get a spouse located in appropriate employment is sometimes essential in bringing a needed professional on board.

Signing bonuses have been popular from time to time during periods of shortage. Currently, it is not unusual to see advertisements for nursing personnel—registered nurses and even support personnel such as nursing assistants—that offer signing bonuses to new employees. A common practice is to pay one-half of the bonus when the person is hired and the second half when the individual has been successfully employed for a period of time, often three to six months.

A frequent practice during shortage periods is to offer a *finder's fee* or *"bounty"* to employees who refer specific candidates who are then hired into shortage occupations. The mechanism for doing so is often referred to as an *employee referral program.* The finder's fee is ordinarily paid out in the same manner as a signing bonus, for example, one-half up front and one-half after the person has remained for a given period of time. It is conceivable that both a signing bonus and a finder's fee can be paid out for getting a single needed position filled. However, there has been evidence suggesting that a sound employee referral program increases in usefulness as the job market tightens and fewer good people are readily available. In spite of the visible costs involved, an employee referral program can save money even when compared with the use of advertising. In many instances a signing bonus and finder's fee together will add up to less than the cost of a modest size display ad placed in a couple of area newspapers. The savings generated by an employee referral program can be significant indeed when compared with the cost of using a search firm. It has often been demonstrated that an employee referral program generates the lowest cost per hire of all recruiting practices.

Generally, hiring managers, executive management, and Human Resources personnel are not eligible for finder's fees. Certain other rules may apply in an employee referral program; for example, an employee will usually be barred from referring a family member or other relative into a job in the referring person's own department. (Most organizations have policies governing the employment of family members.)

Finally, extremely specialized arrangements may be made with individuals who are needed to fill certain critical positions. It is common to hire employed physicians, for example, on the basis of individual personal-service contracts. Another practice occasionally involves an arrangement to pay off an individual's outstanding student loans in exchange for a contractual agreement to remain with the organization for a specific amount of time.

THE SALARY BUMPING GAME

The "salary bumping game" ordinarily involves skilled occupations that are in short supply in a given community or for which the supply in the area is marginal. It begins when a group at one organization applies pressure for more money either by themselves or through an advocate. An advocate may often be a physician whose income depends in part on the occupation in question; for example, an anesthesiologist may advocate on behalf of nurse anesthetists or a surgeon may advocate on behalf of surgical physicians' assistants.

The group or the advocate asks for higher pay for the occupation, citing supposedly higher pay at other organizations in the area and expressing the fear that these better-paying employers are going to lure away some of this group. Some employees may even be "moonlighting" for other employers in the area and may be able to produce "proof" of higher pay at these other places. ("Moonlighters" usually do receive higher hourly rates than regular employees to compensate for the absence of benefits.) The group or the advocate attempts to trade on the fear that the other local employers will take away the best employees unless the group's salaries are increased across the board (that is, for every current employee in the group).

Some organizations will indeed try to lure scarce skills away from other employers in their area, and sometimes they succeed. Pay rates for the occupation in question get bumped upward as organizations recruit each other's people. However, this process does nothing to increase the short supply of the skill in the local area. It does nothing to bring more help into the area; it simply raise personnel costs for all local employers while the shortage persists.

Some professional employees project an attitude of "free agency," that is, they behave as though they are always available to change organizations for what might appear to be a "better deal." These employees probably feel greater loyalty to an occupation or profession than to an organization, and they will move freely, usually for more money, among comparable institutions as long as they feel the professional experience remains about the same from one employer to another. It is the profession that holds them, not any particular organization. As free agents move between organizations they have the effect of bidding up the price for their skills in the community without altering the supply.

The department manager who hears stories to the effect that other local health care employers are or could be threatening to recruit away the best people should first appreciate that this might be true—but it just as likely might be the salary bumping game in action. When hearing such stories, the manager needs to resist the temptation to immediately join the voices calling for more money and do some intelligent investigating. Take the information to Human Resources, which will likely have the means to either verify or refute such claims.

EVERY EMPLOYEE A RECRUITER

Every department manager can have considerable impact on the extent to which the organization appeals to prospective employees. The manager's leadership style and treatment of employees sets the tone for the department and helps create a particular image for that work group. If people within the work group are comfortable in that environment, this shows in their attitude toward working there, and this attitude is visible well beyond the boundaries of the department. If enough departments project this kind of a positive image, the employer will gain a reputation as a good place to work.

Whether there is a referral and reward program in place or not, there is a fundamental truth concerning recruiting: *Whether directly or indirectly, satisfied employees are often an organization's most effective recruiters.*

Discussion Points

1. Explain why it is said that the appropriately operated Human Resources department actually "hires" no one in the sense of selecting a person who will be offered a position.
2. State whether you agree or disagree with this statement, and why: When an employee provides notice of termination or the manager otherwise learns of the employee's impending departure, the manager's very first action should be to submit a requisition for a replacement.
3. Describe at least three important uses of complete and up-to-date job descriptions.
4. Discuss why it is of particular importance in much recruiting activity to begin the search to fill a position by considering persons already within the organization.
5. A colleague of yours who runs a similar department in another local institution telephones you asking for your assess-

ment of a former employee of yours who is applying at his institution. Discuss how much and what kinds of information you should give out.

6. Explain the concept of "negligent hiring" and provide a hypothetical example.

7. Explain the rationale for insisting that checking employment references and providing information in response to reference requests be concentrated at a single point in the organization.

8. Describe the principal hazards in espousing a policy of development from within the organization while aggressively recruiting from the outside.

9. Provide three or four examples of the "free-agent" type of employee and describe the circumstances that at times create free-agent status for them.

10. Explain how employee referral programs, which often include the payment of "signing bonuses" as well as "finder's fees," can often generate the lowest cost-per-hire of all recruiting practices.

CHAPTER 7

How to Conduct a Legal—but Effective— Selection Interview

This chapter—

- Enumerates the specific laws that have implications for the interviewing process
- Reviews recommended preparations for the interviewing manager before the applicant arrives for the interview
- Reviews the interviewing process from the perspective of the interviewing manager
- Reviews in detail the kinds of questions that can and cannot legally be asked in an employment interview
- Offers suggestions about probing for additional information that could be helpful in arriving at an employment decision
- Suggests how the interviewer should respond or react when the applicant voluntarily offers legally forbidden information
- Offers insights into interview behavior, especially concerning applicants who tend to interview the interviewer
- Provides cautionary advice concerning potential fraud and distortion on résumés and applications.

AWASH IN A SEA OF LEGALITIES

Of the laws affecting employment practices (presented in Chapter 3), those that have the most direct effects on interviewing are:

- Title VII of the Civil Rights Act of 1964
- Equal Pay Act of 1963
- Age Discrimination in Employment Act (1967, 1986)

- Americans with Disabilities Act (1992)
- State human rights laws and various local ordinances.

As employment legislation has developed, more and more of what formerly were taken for granted as customary application or interview questions have become illegal. Take a look at an average employment application from the 1970s and compare its contents with the present requirements of law and you will discover that as much as two-thirds of the information requested at that time cannot legally be requested today. These prohibitions extend to interview questioning, specifying what can and cannot legally be asked of a job applicant.

This chapter walks through the entire process from the perspective of a department manager involved in interviewing a prospective employee, from preparation to follow-up. Legal precautions are highlighted as they pertain throughout the process.

BEFORE THE CANDIDATE ARRIVES

In preparation for conducting the interview, the department manager should perform the following activities.

Review the Job Description

Every job description in the department should be reviewed and updated as necessary at regular intervals, perhaps once a year. The department manager should also review the pertinent job description for completeness and accuracy in preparing to interview for an employee to fill that position.

Before interviewing a candidate for the position, the department manager should go through the job description thoroughly and update it as necessary. This should ideally be accomplished as soon as a decision is made that the position will need to be filled. Both the manager and the Human Resources recruiter need the job description early in the process, so if it needs to be updated—or created, in the case of a newly established position—this should be done, and the job description should accompany the personnel requisition to HR.

As the one who supervises the position, you will likely be familiar with many of its characteristics and requirements, but it is just as likely that you may not be able to speak about the position in detail without an up-to-date job description available. If you have many different positions within your responsibility, you may be only generally familiar with the job's structure and requirements.

Review the appropriate job description shortly before the interview is scheduled to occur so that you are thoroughly familiar with the pertinent information about the position. If you need to look up something in the document to answer a question during the interview, fine— but do not lean heavily on the job description during the interview. As manager you are supposed to know about the job and what you will expect of someone in that position.

Review the Application or Résumé

Thoroughly review the individual's job application or résumé before the interview. It does not appear professional to review the application or résumé for the first time in the presence of the applicant, and doing so is bound to be unsettling for the applicant.

Sometimes the interview subject will arrive at your office with résumé or application in hand. If this happens, take just a few minutes in private to go over this material before starting the interview. Human Resources will not ordinarily send the application or résumé along with the applicant unless you are in an urgent recruiting environment in which your organization has agreed to see pertinent applicants on a walk-in basis. Under normal recruiting circumstances you should have the resume or application in advance of the interview; if this is not routine in your organization, discuss the procedure directly with Human Resources.

In reviewing the applicant's information, be especially sensitive to any gaps in the individual's employment record and background. Periods of months or years for which no information is supplied should raise a red flag; such omissions often obscure information the applicant would just as soon not reveal. If you detect gaps, make a note to ask about them during the interview. The Human Resources recruiter should also have looked for gaps in the screening process, but these may not always be detected the first time through.

Be alert also for the possibility of exaggeration and even out-and-out fraud in an applicant's background, especially in the areas of education and work experience. (Résumé fraud will be covered to a greater extent in a later section of this chapter.)

Arrange an Appropriate Time and Place

Arrange for a place to conduct the interview where you and the applicant will be reasonably comfortable and can talk privately. If you have a private office—not an open-top, open-front cubicle, but a complete room with a closable door—use that. If you have no private office—say, for example, you have only a semi-enclosure in the corner of the department—find private space for the interview. Borrow a private office, use a conference room if possible, or ask whether Human Resources can provide space. Whatever kind of area you use, it should always be one in which you can carry on a conversation without being overheard. Trying to conduct an interview within the hearing of others can be distracting for the interviewer and unsettling to the applicant.

Physical comfort is also a consideration. Surroundings need not be plush or elegant, but there should at least be comfortable seating and reasonable temperature control. If you are using a desk or table, position yourself and your visitor so that you are speaking across a corner of the surface or out in an open area rather that across the full expanse of a desk or table. An expanse of surface between you can be intimidating to the applicant.

Make sure to allow adequate time in your schedule for the interview. How long an interview should take depends on the kind of position you are attempting to fill. For entry-level positions perhaps a half-hour may be adequate; for technical and professional positions you may want to allow at least an hour, perhaps even longer should you wish to spend more time with a promising candidate (such as providing a tour of the department).

Plan on keeping the interview completely free from interruptions. Do not take phone calls and do not permit drop-in visitors. Interruptions can disrupt your train of thought and make it difficult for you to establish conversational rapport with the applicant. Make it a rule of interviewing that you want no interruptions short of a true, dire emergency.

Prepare Some Opening Questions

Have a few, perhaps three or four, relatively easy, non-threatening questions ready to get the conversation started. Your review of the person's application or résumé should suggest some simple conversation starters.

CONDUCTING THE ACTUAL INTERVIEW

Taking some basic steps can help you conduct a professional, effective interview. These interview steps are summarized in Exhibit 7-1.

Exhibit 7-1　Tips for the Manager in the Interview Process

- Be on time
- Put the applicant at ease
- Fit your language to the person
- Avoid short-answer questions
- Avoid open-ended questions
- Avoid leading questions
- Keep note-taking to a minimum
- Promise—and ensure—follow-up, but nothing else

Be on Time

You chose the time for the interview, so short of encountering one of those dire emergencies that occur now and then there is no reason for you to be late. If you are indeed late, you should have a plausible (and preferably visible) reason. An employee selection interview is important to the department and should thus be important to you, and it is certainly important to the applicant. Casual tardiness on the interviewer's part displays disregard for the value of the applicant's time, and it can leave the applicant with a less-than-desirable impression of the organization.

Try to Put the Applicant at Ease

Most of the advice we receive about conducting interviews suggests beginning with a bit of small talk, some inconsequential social chatter, to help get the conversation started. With most applicants, this will be enough to get a conversation going. Some applicants are going to remain nervous regardless of whatever you do to encourage them otherwise, but it is still best to make an attempt to put the applicant at ease.

Never lose sight that the applicant may be intimidated by you and the authority of your position. This person knows you are a manager, while he or she remains an outsider looking to be hired into what is probably a nonmanagerial position. To the applicant you are an authority figure who has a strong voice in whether or not he or she gets hired.

As a hiring manager you have the upper hand in the interview situation—the interview is taking place on your home turf, you are a manager, you are a representative of the organization, and you may have the power to extend or withhold employment. Whatever you can do in your approach to put the applicant at ease and carry on the conversation on as equal a footing as possible will help you conduct a more productive interview.

Fit Your Language to the Applicant

Put yourself on the applicant's level of education and sophistication in choosing your words. Speak to the person in terms that he or she is most likely to understand. Unless you know that the applicant is your equivalent in exposure to the work of the department, avoid the use of acronyms without explanation and keep your speech jargon-free, that is, clear of the "inside language" of your field. If you are interviewing personnel for a nursing unit, for example, you will speak with nursing assistant applicants quite differently from the way you speak with registered nurse applicants. This is an important consideration in health care, where the same manager may have direct responsibility for all levels of staff from PhDs down to entry-level support personnel.

Avoid Both Short-Answer Questions and Open-Ended Questions

One of your interview objectives should be to get the individual to talk—about his or her knowledge, experience, reasons for seeking this particular position, likes and dislikes, and career goals. An interviewer will not learn much of substance if the questions can be answered with short answers like "yes," "no," and "three years." Questions should all require the individual to speak at least a sentence or two in response.

Nor should the interviewer ask completely open-ended questions that leave the applicant with no clear idea of what to say or when to stop. A classic example is the opening line so often used by interviewers who believe they are being clever and insightful:

"Tell me about yourself." A question of this nature has no recognizable boundaries, and an answer can ramble on for a considerable time without producing much of value. Moreover, since the question provides no clue as to how much the person is expected to say, it is inherently unfair to the applicant.

The most effective questions are those that require some thought and perhaps two, three, or at the most four sentences to provide a reasonable answer. As an interviewer you should be trying to get the applicant to talk about himself or herself relative to employment, but doing it in such a way that you can maintain control over the conversation and avoid causing the person to either chatter on without end or freeze from confusion when hit with an unfair, open-ended question.

Examples of questions that can elicit the appropriate length and depth of response might include: "How did you become interested in this occupation?" "What part of your most recent position did you like best, and why?" "What accomplishment of the last year or two are you most proud of?" and perhaps "Tell me about something that went wrong on the job and what you learned from it."

Also, be sure to allow a few seconds' pause between an applicant's most recent response and your next question. This gives the individual a chance to tell you more, since most applicants will tend to fill a silence.

Avoid Leading the Applicant

Be careful to avoid leading the applicant toward a response you might want to hear. This is a particular hazard when interviewing someone who is shaping up favorably in your eyes. Often without realizing you are doing so, you begin asking your questions in a manner that encourages the person to provide the answers you want to hear. A sharp applicant will likely pick up on leading questions immediately and will definitely cooperate in coming up with the "right" answers.

Avoid Writing During the Interview

If you must make written reminders for yourself during an interview, limit them to one-or-two word notations. If you feel more detailed notes are required, expand your brief reminders into sentences or paragraphs *after* the interview.

There are two sound reasons for not writing while an applicant is speaking. First, it is unnerving to the applicant because in addition to causing him or her to wonder what you are writing, it restricts eye contact and conveys the impression that you are giving the person less than your complete attention. Second, it is not possible to listen completely and effectively while writing. Few people can perform these two important communication tasks effectively at the same time. It is far better to give the applicant your undivided attention and save the writing until after the interview.

Promise Only Follow-Up

At the conclusion of the interview, indicate to the applicant that he or she will be advised of the outcome after all interviews for the position have been completed and that follow-up will likely come through Human Resources. Promise follow-up, but promise *nothing but* follow-up. Do not promise that an offer will be forthcoming, even if the person you have just interviewed is your leading candidate, and do not presume to make an offer or quote a salary yourself, independent of Human Resources. If the applicant asks specific questions about pay and benefits, refer the person back to the Human Resources recruiter.

Having promised follow-up on behalf of the organization, take steps if you must to ensure that follow-up does occur. Follow-up is ordinarily a Human Resources responsibility, but there is no harm in reminding HR to do it or asking HR whether it has been done. It is extremely important that all applicants who have given their time to the interview process receive closure within some reasonable time following the interview. To allow the unsuccessful applicants to simply fade away without acknowledgment eventually creates ill will toward the employer in the community.

Occasionally an unsuccessful applicant will call the department manager directly and ask specifically why he or she was not hired. Should you receive such a call, you can handle it in one of two ways: You can politely refer the caller to Human Resources for the official response, or you can simply say that the position went to the applicant who seemed best suited for the position. Always be able to defend your reasons for rejecting any particular candidate should it become necessary to do so, but you are under no obligation whatsoever to explain to an unsuccessful applicant why he or she was not the one chosen.

It may be helpful to maintain a brief written record of the reasons for rejecting any particular candidate in a recruiting process, especially if there are a number of applicants involved and your decision might be seen by some as a close or arbitrary call. However, care should be taken regarding what is written and how it is expressed; such notes can "go public" in the event of a legal action stemming from the decision. A good rule of thumb is never write anything to about an applicant that would embarrass you if it appeared in the daily newspaper.

Once again, as department manager you should never involve yourself in checking applicants' references (see Chapter 6). Checking references yourself, going directly to applicants' former bosses, and by-passing the Human Resources departments of both the applicant's former employer and your own organization can easily place you at the center of a legal action.

INTERVIEW QUESTIONING: ASK OR DO NOT ASK?

The days when an interviewer could dig into an applicant's personal life and probe for various personality traits are far behind us. Old ways of questioning probed a great deal toward finding out what the person *is*, while the thrust of present-day—and legal—interviewing is to develop some knowledge of what the person *can do*. As a general rule, keep all interview questions related to the applicant's capabilities to do the job in question.

The following subject areas and commentary offer guidance on what can and cannot legally be asked. Exhibit 7-2 provides specific questions as examples of prohibited inquiries. These questions, or variations of them, may not be asked of a job applicant whether in an interview or on a job application. Exhibit 7-3 provides examples of legal pre-employment interview questions.

There are some legitimate exceptions to the prohibitions against making hiring decisions based on some of these categories of "forbidden information," but not many. For example, there are some instances in which certain factors can legitimately be considered a *bona fide occupational qualification* (BFOQ), such as:

- Gender as a BFOQ, calling only for a male to become a mens' room attendant and only a female to similarly serve a ladies' room, or hiring females only to model womens' clothing and males only to model mens' clothing
- Possession of a *driver's license* as a BFOQ for a position that requires driving for the employer.

Race or Color, Religion or Creed, National Origin, Sex, Marital Status, Birth Control Practices

There are *no questions* concerning these subject areas that can legally be asked. This means no questions about the origins of the person's name, where the person's family came from, or even whether the person has a family at all. No questions about any of these are permitted, and that goes as well for peripheral questions that can be interpreted as "fishing"

Exhibit 7-2   Examples of Forbidden Pre-Employment Questions

General
1. Do you attend church regularly? What church do you go to, and who is the pastor?
2. What religious holidays do you observe?
3. What is your nationality, ancestry, descent, parentage, lineage, etc.?
4. What nationality are your parents? Your spouse?
5. What is your native language?
6. Are you married? Divorced? Separated?
7. Where does your spouse work? What does he (or she) do for a living?
8. Do you have children? What are their names and ages? Do you have a reliable arrangement for child care?
9. When were you born? How old are you?
10. Was your name ever changed by marriage or court order? If so, what was your original name?
11. Where were you born?
12. Where were your parents born? Where was your spouse born?
13. Of what country are you a citizen?
14. Are you a native-born or naturalized citizen of the United States?
15. Do you own your own home, or do you rent?
16. How did you acquire the ability to read, write, or speak fluently?
17. What is the name, address, and relationship to you of the individual to be notified in case of accident or emergency?
18. What kind of discharge did you receive from the U.S. military?
19. To what clubs, societies, lodges, or fraternal organizations do you belong?
20. How many children do you plan to have?
21. Have you ever had your wages garnished or attached?
22. Have you ever filed bankruptcy, either personally or as a business owner?
23. Has your spouse ever worked here?
24. What is your height? Your weight?
25. Would your spouse approve of your employment here should you be hired?

Medical:
Concerning an applicant's medical history, in a pre-employment interview the employer may not:
• Ask a general question to determine if the applicant has any disabilities (medical or physical limitation) that could prevent the person from performing the duties of the job in question

continues

Exhibit 7-2 Examples of Forbidden Pre-Employment Questions (continued)

- Ask about medical history or work-related accidents, or ask the applicant to check off on a list of potentially disabling physical impairments that he or she may have
- Ask about the applicant's worker's compensation history, if any
- Ask how an applicant became disabled or inquire into the prognosis concerning a specific disability
- Ask whether the applicant will require time off for treatment or medical leave due to anticipated incapacitation because of a disability.

Some specific examples of questions about medical or physical status that cannot legally be asked are:

1. Are you in any way disabled, or do you have a disability?
2. Have you ever filed a worker's compensation claim?
3. Have you ever been injured at work?
4. Will you require time off for medical reasons?
5. Is any member of your family disabled?
6. Do you have any medical, physical, or mental disorder that could prevent you from performing the duties of the job?
7. Have you ever been hospitalized? For what conditions?
8. Are you taking prescription medication? What drugs, prescribed for what conditions?
9. If you are presently out of work because of a disability, what is the prognosis?
10. Have you or any member of your family ever been treated for any of the following diseases or disabilities? (There follows a checkoff list that may include: cancer, heart disease, high blood pressure, diabetes, epilepsy, AIDS, back problems, carpal tunnel syndrome, hearing loss, contact dermatitis, hearing loss, drug or alcohol abuse, arthritis, tendonitis, and perhaps numerous additional ailments.)

for forbidden information. Note also that it is illegal to request any of this information on an employment application.

The reasoning behind these prohibitions is of course the possibility of discrimination based on such information. For example, at one time it was common to ask young female applicants if they were engaged and if so when they planned to marry, to ask married women if they had or planned to have children, and to ask divorced or separated women if they were single parents and how many children they had.

Exhibit 7-3 Examples of Legally Permissible Pre-Employment Questions

1. What is your full name?
2. What is your address and the telephone number at which you can be reached?
3. What is your prior work experience? For each prior employer this may include:
   - employer's name and address
   - jobs or positions held
   - duties performed
   - skills needed to perform job duties
   - tools, machinery, equipment, and vehicles used in job performance
   - name of immediate supervisor
   - rate of pay received
   - length of time on the job
   - reasons for leaving.
4. What skills, education, training, or experience have you had that is relevant to the performance of the duties of this job?
5. Are you able to work the particular shift(s) on which this job is ordinarily performed?
6. Are you able to work overtime or weekends when necessary?
7. Are you able to meet this organization's attendance standard?
8. If hired, when would you be able to begin work?
9. Are you applying for full-time, part-time, temporary, etc., work?
10. Do you hold the licenses or certifications that may be required for employment in the position in question (e.g., driver's license, electrician's license, registered nursing license).
11. What were your primary duties and most important responsibilities on your most recent job?
12. What do you know about the requirements of the job for which you are applying?
13. What do you believe was the most difficult part of the job you have been most recently doing? Why?
14. What safety procedures were you required to follow at your most recent employment?

Information obtained in answer to such questions was used to make hiring decisions, with many managers believing it was simply good business to try to avoid hiring people who might not remain in their jobs very long or who might experience more absences than others who lacked certain responsibilities.

Anti-discrimination legislation has deemed it illegal to make employment decisions based on personal information, leading to today's essential focus on determining to the extent possible what the individual is capable of doing.

Age

Essentially the only legal question an applicant can be asked about age is: Are you at least 18 years of age? It is permissible, at times even necessary, to ask this because the employment of workers younger than 18 is governed by most states' child labor laws, and there are numerous employment circumstances prohibited for those under 18.

For the most part, the prohibitions on questions about age relate to age discrimination laws, and age can be considered a legitimate employment criterion only in those relatively few circumstances when it is a BFOQ (see Chapter 3 for examples). In the vast majority of employment situations age cannot be regarded as a qualification; again, the single criterion that prevails is the individual's ability to do the job.

Disability

The Americans with Disabilities Act (ADA) prohibits an employer from asking whether an applicant has a disability or has ever been treated for any number of specific medical conditions. The employer is also forbidden to ask about an applicant's worker's compensation history any time prior to making an offer of employment. All that can be asked during the pre-offer stage of the employment process are questions concerning the person's ability to perform the functions of the job. Questions asked at this stage cannot be phrased such that they actually solicit information about medical conditions or physical limitations. For example, if a job requires driving, the interviewer may ask if the applicant has a driver's license but may not ask if the person has any visual limitation.

In inquiring into an applicant's ability to perform the major functions of the job, the interviewer can ask if the person has any impairment (medical, physical, or mental) that could interfere with his or her ability to do the job, or whether there are any kinds of positions the person should not be considered for because of some impairment. It is illegal, however, for the interviewer to ask about the nature of the impairment. The key to questioning in this area is to focus on ability, not disability.

Name

It is permissible for the interviewer to ask whether the individual has ever worked for this organization under a different name; the employer is entitled to know to be able to access the individual's prior work record. One may also ask whether there is any additional information concerning a name change or use of a different name that may be needed to accomplish reference checks.

However, the interviewer is forbidden to ask a female applicant's maiden name or the original name of an applicant whose name has been changed by court order.

Address and Duration of Residence

It is permissible to ask an applicant's place of residence and how long the person has been a resident of this municipality.

Birthplace and Date of Birth

There are no questions that can legally be asked concerning an applicant's place of birth or that of the applicant's parents or any other family members, and it is illegal in most instances to ask the applicant's age. Also illegal is a practice formerly engaged in by a number of employers requiring the applicant to submit a birth certificate, baptismal record, naturalization record, or other proof of age.

Photograph

The practice of some employers of years past requiring an applicant to supply a photograph with his or her application is illegal, as is even suggesting that a photograph may be submitted at the individual's option.

Citizenship

It is lawful to ask whether an applicant is a citizen of the United States, but unlawful to ask of what country the individual is a citizen (such is construed as asking for national origin). One who is not a citizen can legally be asked whether he or she intends to become one or has the legal right to remain and work in the United States. It is also legal to require the applicant to state whether he or she has ever been arrested or interned as an enemy alien.

On the illegal side, it is not permissible to ask whether an applicant or the applicant's parents or spouse are naturalized or native-born U.S. citizens, and an applicant cannot be required to produce naturalization papers.

Language

It is legal to ask what foreign languages an applicant is able to speak and write fluently. However, it is not legal to ask an individual his or her native language or to ask how the person acquired the ability to read, speak, or write a foreign language.

Education

It is legal to ask about an applicant's academic, vocational, or professional education and the public or private schools the person attended, including discussion of the relevance of particular programs or courses taken.

Experience

This is the area in which much of the interviewer's questioning should be concentrated. Your primary objective in this phase of the interview process should be to gather sufficient information about the applicant's work history to allow you to judge whether the individual's experience is applicable to the position you are attempting to fill.

In talking about employment experience, it is usually most helpful to begin with the applicant's present or most recent position and work backward in time.

Relatives

It is permissible to ask the names of the applicant's relatives (other than spouse) who are already employed within your organization. It is illegal to solicit any information concerning the applicant's spouse, children, or other relatives who are not employed by your organization.

Whom to Notify in Case of Emergency

In the pre-employment stage of recruiting it is illegal to ask an applicant for the name and address of a person to be notified in the event of accident or other emergency. This is one of the elements of information (along with date of birth, marital and family status, and other personal information) the organization is not permitted to solicit until an offer of employment has been extended and accepted.

Military Experience

It is permissible to ask about the nature of an applicant's military experience in a branch of the armed forces of the United States. However, one may not ask about general military experience (without specifying armed forces of the United States or a branch thereof), and it is not permissible to ask an applicant about the character of his or her discharge or separation from military service (honorable, general, medical, dishonorable, etc.).

Arrest

Although "Have you ever been arrested?" was essentially a standard question on applications and in interviews for many years, it is no longer legal. It is, however, permissible to ask if one has ever been *convicted* of a crime, and to ask for the details associated with the conviction.

Information acquired from this question must be used with care. If an individual is rejected for employment because of a criminal conviction, there should be a reasonable relationship between the nature of the crime and the position for which the person is applying. For example, the organization may be acting properly and reasonably in rejecting a convicted embezzler for a finance position or rejecting someone with a drug-related conviction for a pharmacy position, but may encounter claims of discrimination for rejecting someone with a felony DWI conviction for a position as a cook or housekeeper.

Organizations

Another age-old common request asked applicants to "List all clubs, societies, and other organizations to which you belong." This is now illegal, since the very names of many organizations allow one to infer personal information such as national origin or religion.

One absolute prohibition concerning external memberships involves inquiries into whether the applicant is or ever has been a member of a labor union. Employers, especially those who may be union-free, ordinarily do not want to knowingly bring on board someone they fear might attempt to spread interest in union organizing. Past years have seen numerous instances of applicants claiming they were rejected for employment because of union affiliations.

To remain legal, an inquiry about organizations must be limited to asking about membership in organizations the applicant considers relevant to his or her ability to handle the position. For all practical purposes this limits questions about organizations to technical and professional societies related to one's occupational field.

PROBING FOR INTANGIBLES

After discussing the more concrete subjects such as qualifications and experience with the applicant, it can be helpful for the interviewer to spend some time discussing less tangible areas and attempting to develop an overall impression of the person and his or her attitude toward work and careers. Since there is so much that cannot be asked in an interview, it is now more important than ever to develop a "gut feel" for the candidate. Certainly this is highly subjective, but it is also a legitimate part of the interview process—the feeling you develop about an individual during an interview can be a forerunner of how you come to regard that person as an employee.

Exhibit 7-4 offers a number of possible questions that can be used in assessing the applicant in areas other than specific qualifications and ex-

---

Exhibit 7-4 Examples of Questions to Use in Probing the Intangibles

1. What aspects of a job are most important to you?
2. What are your own personal criteria for your success?
3. What are your short-term career goals? Long-term career goals?
4. What are you looking for here that you are not getting from your present position?
5. What past goals have you set for yourself, and what have you done to accomplish them?
6. In what way would a position with our organization help meet your growth?
7. What factors do you believe have contributed the most to your growth?
8. What has prevented you from moving ahead as rapidly as you would have liked?
9. What job would you choose if you were completely free to do so?
10. Which of your jobs did you enjoy the most? Why?
11. How did you get each of the positions you held?

perience. In addition to assessing the intangibles, the interviewer should keep another question in mind throughout the conversation: How well do I believe this person would fit into the present work group? Whoever you hire will have to work with your current employees day in and day out, perhaps quite closely. It is certainly legitimate for you to be considering how this particular personality might relate to those already there.

While assessing the intangibles, and perhaps throughout the interview overall, the interviewer should be attempting to judge whether this applicant, in interviewing for the job you are attempting to fill, is trying to obtain something desired or escape something dissatisfying. In others words, you are trying to determine whether the applicant's driving force is positive—that is, the person is seeking advancement, more interesting work, a preferred occupation, growth or personal satisfaction, or more attractive compensation. In contrast, the applicant's driving force may be negative—trying to get away from an unpleasant environment, undesirable hours, an unpleasant supervisor, or a quarrelsome mix of personalities.

It is not always easy to determine whether the person's motivations in seeking the position are positive, negative, or mixed; nonetheless, it is worth the time to consider. The person who is seeking something desired is more likely to remain a positive performer over the longer term, while the one whose primary motive is to escape something is more likely to be a mediocre performer who becomes another turnover statistic before too long.

WHEN FORBIDDEN INFORMATION IS VOLUNTEERED

Forbidden information should never be used as the basis of an employment decision, even when it is given to you voluntarily.

Anyone who has conducted at least a few employee selection interviews has probably received so-called forbidden information at one time or another. This of course puts the interviewing manager somewhat on the spot; you have heard what you did not ask for and what you are not supposed to know. You must ignore the information, but doing so is usually easier said than done. The situation is similar to that we hear so frequently in courtroom dramas. An objection is offered and sustained, following which the judge might say, "The jury is to disregard that last remark." It is not easy to disregard something we have heard, however. The best we can often do is to conscientiously avoid factoring that information into our decision.

An applicant will often volunteer personal information in what amounts to a plea for sympathy that will lead to a job offer. At one time or another most interviewers have heard statements like, "I really need this job because I'm a single parent," "I've been out of work for months and my husband is ill," or "We get our health insurance through my wife's employer, so I could save you some money on benefits."

On occasion it also happens that someone will drop an item of personal information quite deliberately, then later claim discrimination when the job goes to someone else: "I happened to mention that I was pregnant—I know that's why I didn't get the job."

To reiterate, no matter how it is obtained, so-called forbidden information should never be used as a factor in an employment decision. But since it is also possible to be required to defend any particular employment decision, the hiring manager should always be able to state succinctly and honestly why one person was hired in preference to other.

THE INTERVIEWER'S BEHAVIOR

Occasionally employee selection interviews become interviews of *you* and thus of the organization. Some applicants seem to do this naturally, and there are some undeniably sharp applicants who can deliberately turn the focus of an interview from them to the interviewer.

More Silence Than Talk

Some interviewers tend to dominate the conversation, carrying on at length about the organization, their departments, and often themselves. The object of the interview is to get the applicant to talk about himself or herself, and specifically to talk about appropriately job-related topics. The interviewer must control the interview with the proper questioning and concentrate on what the applicant is saying. The proper role of the interviewer involves more silence than speech; from the interviewer's perspective, the most productive parts of an interview occur with the mouth shut and the ears open.

Non-stop talking by the interviewer limits the information that can be gained from the applicant and also sends the applicant an inappropriate message about the organization.

More Points to Keep in Mind

Effective interviewing involves being in complete control of the interview situation without obviously appearing to do so.

At all times try to resist the temptation to rush to judgment concerning a job candidate. Many interviewers make up their minds about candidates during the first few minutes of contact, and the remainder of the interview does little to change that mindset. Always keep in mind that even though first impressions are sometimes proven correct, just as often they are proven incorrect.

Never encourage an applicant to criticize a present or past employer, and be wary of the applicant who voluntarily does so. On the other hand, one indicator of a promising applicant can be how diplomatically the individual describes what seems to have been an unpleasant employment experience.

Remain aware of the non-verbal clues that an interviewee may exhibit during the course of the interview, although you should allow for normal nervousness, especially with applicants who are new to interviewing.

Be conscious of the "halo effect" in interviewing. This occurs when the interviewer allows one or two obviously positive traits to favorably bias his or her judgment on unrelated characteristics.

In every interview try to convey an overall positive picture of the organization. If you project the belief that the organization is a good place to work, some of this positive view will be communicated to the applicant.

Be honest about the negatives of the job, if any. Many jobs have a downside, and some include decidedly unappealing tasks or situations. Remain upbeat overall, but do not overlook the negatives during the interview process; an applicant who accepts a position only to discover the unpleasant parts after starting work is likely to feel that he or she has not been dealt with honestly.

RÉSUMÉ FRAUD: LIES AND EMBELLISHMENTS

At times it seems that the writing of employment résumés involves putting nearly as much fiction as fact on paper. It has been estimated that up to 40 percent of résumés include exaggerations or outright untruths, and perhaps as many as 75 percent include some degree of "puff," making facts appear more significant than they may actually be by putting a favorable spin on them.

Deception on employment résumés can take a number of different forms, including:

- *Deliberate ambiguity.* One of the most frequently encountered instances of this has to do with education. An individual will claim to have "*attended* Prestige University in the BS Program in Chemistry," hoping that the reader will automatically assume graduation and receipt of the degree.
- *Deliberate shifting of dates* of education or experience to conceal a period of unemployment, or occasionally a period of imprisonment. An honest résumé may show a gap, and many applicants know that gaps in their records will be questioned.
- *Using years only* to create the impression of having worked longer in a place than was actually the case, for example, stating one worked for "Ajax Hospital, 2000-2001" hoping the reader will assume two years when it may actually have been November 2000 through January 2001. The years-only ploy is also used to hide gaps in employment.
- *Exaggerated job responsibilities,* inflated job titles, and inflated salaries, all intended to make the applicant look more appealing than might otherwise be the case.
- *Claims of a "better" school* awarding one's degree. For example, Applicant X holds an MBA from obscure Nowhere University, but X's résumé describes it as a "Harvard MBA."
- *False claims of degrees and other credentials,* and inflated or invented honors, awards, conference presentations, and publications.

Résumé fraud understandably increases during periods of job scarcity. However, it is present to some extent on a continuing basis, so employment recruiters and other interviewers should be alert to the possibility of fraud in every résumé they review.

There is no way to reliably uncover every instance of fraud, exaggeration, or untruth that may appear in the résumés the organization receives. It would be prohibitively time-consuming and costly to verify every claim on a résumé. However, interviewers can remain alert to certain signs and signals that could mean some closer examination is warranted:

- Always look for *gaps* in the person's record. It is common for someone who wants to cover up something to simply omit it.
- Be alert for *overlapping dates and inconsistent details.* An untruth here and there can upset the chronology of one's experience, and

the person fudging the facts often fails to adjust other information as necessary.

- Ask some *questions about the prestigious school* the applicant claims to have attended or the city in which the applicant claims to have worked. Many of those who have put themselves in the position of "making it up as they go along" will fumble, stumble, or hesitate in coming up with answers.

- Always consider an applicant's *reason for leaving* a particular position and ask for clarification, especially if the job sought actually represents a downward or even lateral move. Most people who have been terminated from a job for cause (not laid off, but fired) will use wording that characterizes their departures as voluntary.

- Question the applicant about *specific details* that appear in the résumé. The person who has lied or exaggerated will often find it more difficult to remember everything that he or she wrote.

- Try to decide whether the job candidate's *answers seem memorized or rehearsed.* Someone with nothing to conceal does not need to have pat answers prepared in advance.

- Always be conscious of *nonverbal clues.* Excessive nervousness, failure to look you in the eye, or fidgeting in the chair can sometimes be indicators of fraud.

- Ask the individual for *permission to have specific information verified.* The applicant who has faked something significant may well withdraw from the process right after the interview.

Human Resources will frequently become involved in verifying résumé information. This is of course what is being done when work references are checked, but sometimes verification has to go beyond ordinary reference checks. When confirming information by telephone the HR representative will go through a company's operator or Human Resources department rather than using a telephone number the applicant may have provided. Some who fake their experience have friends or relatives pose as former employers. Also, if there is any doubt about whether a reference's address is genuine, HR will test the address by mailing something there.

AN ACQUIRED SKILL

Many who are new to management are initially uneasy about interviewing prospective employees. This uneasiness often make the interviewing process more difficult than it needs to be.

The department manager who takes interviewing seriously, conscientiously tries to do it effectively, and endeavors to learn from each interview experience will find that interviewing skill improves with practice. Being too casual and disorganized in interviewing can cause you to lose a potentially good hire and leave that person with a poor impression of the organization. On the other hand, being too careful, dragging out the process by interviewing numerous people, and delaying a decision can also result in the loss of a potentially good employee.

It helps to remember that when it comes to selecting employees, there is no guaranteed perfect choice. There is always some risk. It is often said that the personal interview is a problematic and not especially reliable means of filling a job—but there is no better means available.

Discussion Points

1. In interviewing a prospective employee, explain why you should you consider it important to inquire into information gaps—time periods unaccounted for—in the applicant's work record.
2. Explain why the interviewing manager should review all available information about an applicant before beginning an interview? Managers are busy people—should it not be sufficient for the applicant to arrive for an interview with application in hand?
3. In an employment interview, the interviewer should want the applicant to do most of the talking. Explain what is wrong with opening with: "Tell me all about yourself."
4. Provide three examples of interview questions that are legal but that provide the interviewing manager with little or no useful information.
5. Explain why it is no longer appropriate to ask whether a job applicant has ever been arrested. Is it not in the employer's best interests to avoid taking on workers who have run afoul of the law?
6. Discuss whether or not you can make use of personal information in rendering an employment decision if the information was provided to you voluntarily. Why, or why not?
7. State whether you agree or disagree with this statement, and why: The interviewing manager should be prepared to respond

in considerable detail to any unsuccessful job candidate who calls asking why he or she was not offered employment.

8. Discuss why it is often said that the proper role of the interviewer involves more silence than speech.

9. Develop a brief procedure or protocol—a simple list of points—for reviewing an employment application or résumé for possible inaccuracies or embellishments.

10. Write—or quote from somewhere in the chapter—one concise statement which, if always conscientiously applied in interviewing, will practically ensure that all questions asked will be legal.

11. Explain why it is important for the interviewing manager to attempt to assess an applicant relative to intangible factors not directly reflected in a record of education or experience.

12. Discuss why it is advisable to keep writing to a minimum while interviewing an applicant. Shouldn't a manager try to capture as much information as possible about the person?

PART IV

Employee Relations and the Manager

CHAPTER 8

Directions in Employee Relations

This chapter—

- Describes the evolution of employee relations through three distinct philosophies: authoritarian, legalistic, and humanistic
- Discusses the emergence of "scientific management" and the development of other means of organizing and managing human enterprise
- Examines opposing assumptions about people that influence various approaches to management, and briefly reviews theories of human motivation
- Reviews the growth of official government concern for the social welfare of American workers
- Projects the likely direction of labor relations for the coming years.

THE EVOLUTION OF EMPLOYEE RELATIONS

From the beginnings of organized work activity, when one person first directed the work of others, employee relations seems to have evolved through three identifiable philosophies of management: authoritarian, legalistic, and humanistic.

Authoritarian employee relations arose first, followed much later by legalistic and humanistic employee relations. One is still able to find organizations that operate on what is essentially an authoritarian philosophy, although pure authoritarianism is rare in American business and is steadily becoming even more rare. We can find many organizations in which the legalistic philosophy prevails, and a number of organizations in which the humanistic philosophy is gradually replacing the others.

Authoritarian Management

Authoritarian management goes back to the beginnings of organized enterprise, perhaps even back to the first master-slave relationship. Authoritarian management takes a rather dim view of people, seemingly operating on the assumption that for the most part people have to be continually told what to do to obtain the best possible output. Authoritarian management was the generally accepted form for centuries; the boss gave orders and expected them to be carried out.

This is not to suggest that authoritarian management is always harsh or cruel. Certainly the authoritarian manager is autocratic, but autocratic types can vary greatly. At one end of the spectrum is the exploitative autocrat (from the "the Attila-the-Hun school of management"), generally the cruel leader who quite literally exploits his followers for personal gain. At the opposite end of the spectrum is the benevolent autocrat. The benevolent autocrat (from the "father-knows-best school of management") looks after his followers and sees that they are protected and well cared for—as long as they do exactly as they are told, without question. Regardless of which end of the spectrum he or she may be coming from, the autocratic manager calls all the shots and gives all the orders, and the followers can do as they are told—or leave.

Many people now in the work force have worked under strongly authoritarian managers and some do so even today. However, authoritarianism steadily diminished during the twentieth century, especially during the second half, and continues to diminish during these early years of the twenty-first century.

For many years the authoritarian manager's style was essentially to do as he or she wished. For a long while employees had very few legal rights, so managers could manage as they pleased with little regard for resistance and little fear of legal repercussions. But then legalism intruded.

Legalistic Management

The legalistic movement took root with wage and hour laws and labor laws in the 1930s, blossomed with passage of the Civil Rights Act of 1964, and has ever since been fed by a nearly steady stream of legislation addressing employment and employee rights (see Chapter

3). Strictly authoritarian management had to adjust, although not always readily or willingly, to the accumulating legal restrictions.

Managers began to treat people differently, and generally better, than they had under purely authoritarian management primarily because the law was now telling them what they could or could not do. This legalistic phase of employee relations has been shaped, defined, and bounded by legislation. We find managers dealing with employees out of a strict regard for employees' rights—not because they realize it is the right thing to do, but rather because they want to keep themselves and their employers out of legal trouble. Legalistic employee relations brought the outlook of the bureaucrat to some managers in that regulations began to take precedence over people.

Humanistic Management

Two significant areas of influence have contributed to the growth of humanistic management: (1) the still-expanding structure of legislation that essentially mandated humane treatment of employees, and (2) the lasting effects of the human relations movement in management that has been growing and developing since the middle of the twentieth century. This movement essentially recognized employees' rights before they became legally mandated and fostered the belief that contented, well-treated employees who were dealt with fairly and equitably were generally better producers and more loyal employees than those who were not so well regarded.

There is one area of essential difference between legalistic management and humanistic management: The legalistic manager behaves in a certain manner because that is what the law requires, while the humanistic manager behaves in that manner because he or she believes that it is right and proper to do so. Legalistic management may continue to be driven in part by some pessimistic and somewhat authoritarian assumptions about people, while humanistic management holds the optimistic view that satisfied workers produce best.

The progression from authoritarian to legalistic to humanistic management can be simplistically described as the progression from pushing people to directing people to leading people.

Residual Authoritarianism

If we know why the laws addressing employee rights are to be respected and obeyed, and if we believe that satisfied employees are better producers, why do we continue to see noticeable authoritarianism in management in so many places? Consider that for many, many years, in fact for centuries, autocratic management was essentially the only management style. Deeply ingrained into the population's overall view of management were such concepts as the giving of orders, the bearing of responsibility, the making of decisions, and the placement or removal of people as needed or desired. Management was authoritarianism largely by definition.

Next consider: How have most managers traditionally learned about management? A growing number of managers now learn some of the basics of management in formal education programs but find it necessary to absorb most of what they learn on the job, through their management role models. Not long ago, however, essentially all managers learned by emulating their role models, and their role models learned from *their* role models, who in turn learned from role models who were authoritarian in outlook and practice. Thus a strain of authoritarianism, weakening with each subsequent generation of managers but still present, has been passed down the line to today's managers. In some respects human behavior changes slowly, especially in a pursuit such as management in which old beliefs and attitudes have had hundreds of years in which to solidify.

THE EMERGENCE OF SCIENTIFIC MANAGEMENT

Undoubtedly authoritarianism in employee relations was aided, prolonged, and even intensified in places by the emergence of what became known as "scientific management." In the early years of the twentieth century there was a movement toward the scientific study of business management activities with an orientation toward making them as efficient as possible. A number people figured prominently in this movement, including Frederick W. Taylor, Henry L. Gantt, Frank Bunker, Frank and Lillian Gilbreth, and others. These pioneers of "scientific management" were largely responsible for the original shape of the field of industrial engineering.

Scientific management seemed to intensify authoritarianism and sustain its existence in some business pursuits, especially manufacturing. It was extremely unpopular in some quarters, and it was indeed evident that by reducing work to simple segments and repetitive methods the focus was clearly far more on process and production than on people. A November 1913 resolution of the American Federation of

Labor (AFL) referred to the "Taylor system" as "a diabolical scheme for the reduction of the human being to the condition of a mere machine."[1]

Taylor and his colleagues settled early on the term "scientific management" to describe their organized approach to proceduralizing work, standardizing methods, and improving productivity. It was scientific management that gave American industry assembly lines and other repetitive work situations and strengthened the concept of production-centered management.

PARALLEL MANAGEMENT SYSTEMS DEVELOP

Two systems or approaches to management appear to have developed in parallel during the early decades of the twentieth century, one in activities in which repetitive work is dominant and the other in activities in which varied work prevails. These systems were described by Rensis Likert as the job *organization system* and the *cooperative motivation system.*[2]

In Likert's job organization system repetitive work is dominant. Jobs are usually well organized, with considerable structure to them such that extremely specific job descriptions are possible (think of the job description of an assembly line worker). Tight controls are possible; output can be scheduled with considerable accuracy, inputs to the processes can likewise be scheduled to feed into the system when and where they are needed, and overall the speed of a process can be set and maintained at a predictable level. In a properly designed process under the job organization system inefficiencies are held to a minimum and remain well under control. The approach to management is ordinarily advanced and well organized.

Management within the job organization system is decidedly production-centered, with the focus on the process and its output. It is the system that moves the people, or rather it is the people who are carried along with the system. Picture an assembly line. The line runs at a set speed, and the people keep up with it. If one person is not available to serve the line, another is plugged into that spot and the line continues to move. What keeps the line moving, what keeps the wheels turning in any variation of the job organization system, is the economic motivations of the workers—people coming to work because they are paid to do so. The very functioning of the job organization system is dependent on economic motives. It was essentially the work of Taylor and the other proponents of scientific management that gave us the job organization system.

In Likert's cooperative motivation system it is varied work that prevails. Most jobs are loosely organized, with such a variety of possible activities and responsibilities that job descriptions are necessarily all-encompassing and decidedly non-specific (think of the job description of a registered nurse). Tight controls are not possible; output cannot be scheduled except in the most vague and general terms. Some secondary inputs to the processes can perhaps be scheduled reasonably well but in many instances the primary inputs (in health care, think patients) come into the system with unpredictable frequency, and in most instances the speed of a process cannot be maintained at a predictable level. The approach to management is not well organized, requiring the regular exercise of judgment and impromptu decision-making.

Management within the cooperative motivation system is necessarily people-centered, with the focus on the human elements (in health care, both worker and patient). It is the people who move the system; the system fails to function if the people do not make it happen. Picture an emergency room. Given the nature of the cases encountered, the pace with which the process functions is up to the workers. If one person is not available to work an assigned job, the entire process has to adjust to account for the missing person and efficiency and output suffer. In any variation of the cooperative motivation system it is the people who keep the system moving, people coming to work not only because they are paid to do so but also because they are willing to do so. The very functioning of the cooperative motivation system is dependent on individual enthusiasm and motivation.

Management that is inclined toward authoritarianism is more likely to encounter only nominal resistance within the job organization system. It may engender resentment and foster something of an adversarial relationship between workers and management, but since many of the workers will be fully as production-centered as management, they will expect and to some extent accept being management's secondary focus after output.

Carry management that is inclined toward authoritarianism into the environment of a cooperative motivation system, and the results are ordinarily less than satisfactory. Most of health care falls under the cooperative motivation system, making it far more amenable to people-centered management than production-centered management. With this essential focus on people, the humanistic philosophy of employee relations becomes all the more important.

Exhibit 8-1 compares the characteristics of the job organization system and the cooperative motivation system.

An Opposing View of Employees

One of the individuals whose work contributed much to the human relations movement in management was Douglas McGregor. In his classic paper, "The Human Side of Enterprise," McGregor gave us a readily understandable continuum of assumptions about people as applied to work activity in the form of his *Theory* X and *Theory* Y.[3]

Within both Theory X and Theory Y, it is assumed that management is responsible for organizing and applying the elements of productive enterprise, that is, money and thus equipment, materials, and people. However, this is as far as the similarity between X and Y goes.

Theory X assumes that without active management intervention to direct their efforts, motivate them, control their actions, and modify their behavior to fit the needs of the organization, employees are indifferent, passive, and even resistant to organizational needs. This pessimistic view of employees holds that employees must be persuaded to do what is needed, rewarded for doing proper things right, punished for doing wrong, and in general be controlled as needed.

The underlying assumptions of Theory X are that:

- The average person is indolent by nature, working as little as possible
- Most people lack ambition, dislike responsibility, and prefer to be led

Exhibit 8-1 Job Organization System versus Cooperative Motivation System

Characteristic	Job Organization	Cooperative Motivation
Dominant Work	Repetitive	Variable
Job Structure	More Rigid	Looser
Controllability of System	Greater	Lesser
Output Predictability	Greater	Lesser
Primary System Drivers	Economic	Personal Willingness
Nature of Management	Production-Centered	People-Centered

- When people become employees they remain self-centered and generally indifferent to organizational needs
- People are by nature resistant to change
- The average person is gullible, easily duped, and not particularly bright.

Theory X can be "hard" in its applications, involving coercion, threats, punishment, close supervision, and tight controls on behavior. On the other hand, X can be "soft" in its applications, being permissive, satisfying people's demands, and giving employees what they want to get them to be tractable, accept direction, and produce as desired. Whether hard or soft, however, the unflattering assumptions about people remain the same.

Also, Theory X, whether hard or soft, is inadequate to motivate employees because the human needs on which it relies are unimportant as motivators of human behavior.

Theory Y represents the other end of the continuum, the direct opposite of Theory X. The underlying assumptions of Theory Y are:

- People are *not* by nature passive or resistant to organizational needs; if they appear to be so, they have become this way through experience in organizations
- The motivation, capacity, potential, and readiness to work toward organizational goals are present in all people; management cannot put these into people but is responsible for helping people recognize and develop these characteristics
- Management must arrange conditions so that people can best achieve their goals by directing their own efforts toward organizational objectives.

McGregor's work included a hierarchy of human needs parallel to that described by A. H. Maslow in "A Theory of Human Motivation."[4] Both McGregor and Maslow advanced the notion that humans are constantly in search of need satisfaction and that when a need at one level is satisfied, another, higher-order, need arises to take its place. The need hierarchies of McGregor and Maslow are essentially the same:

- At the most fundamental level are *physiological needs*, the need for air, food, water, etc. Both McGregor and Maslow used the same name for this level.

- Next are *safety needs*, the need for protection from harm, for shelter. Again, both used the same name.
- Progressing from safety needs, next encountered are what McGregor called *social needs* and Maslow called *love needs*. By either name, this represents the need to belong, the need for acceptance, the need for inclusion in groups (work organization, family, clubs, etc.).
- At the next level are what McGregor called *ego needs* and Maslow called *psychological needs*. These include the need for praise and reward or recognition, for accomplishment, for satisfaction in work, and in general the need to feel good about one's self.
- At the ultimate level are what McGregor referred to as *self-fulfillment needs* and what Maslow called *self-actualization*. Again, these are essentially the same, representing the ultimate in need satisfaction, which we might briefly describe as doing or being that which brings the individual ultimate personal fulfillment and satisfaction.

Inherent in the work of both McGregor and Maslow is the belief that a satisfied need is not a motivator of behavior. In this day and age, for a great many people most of the time the physiological, safety, and social needs are met. When this is the case, individuals are then found to be striving to fulfill psychological or ego needs—they want to accomplish and achieve, to acquire competence, to acquire knowledge, to secure recognition and appreciation, and so on. The lower-order needs prevail only when a person has suffered some form of deprivation and gone "backward" in the hierarchy. For example, an individual who is out of work and running out of money with which to secure the basics of life (that is, to fulfill physiological and safety needs) doubtless has securing a job as first priority and at that time is not much concerned with social or psychological needs. As quoted in McGregor's landmark paper, "Man lives by bread alone, when there is no bread."

LONG-TERM TRENDS IN ORGANIZATIONAL MANAGEMENT

Two long-terms trends dominated management during the twentieth century. First, introduced more than 100 years ago, was scientific management. It had considerable influence on management practices, but as suggested earlier, even though it brought improvements in productivity, it also had adverse effects on the human side of organizational activity.

The other trend began shortly following the end of World War I when social scientists began taking a critical look at the negative fallout of scientific management. This was the beginning of the *human relations movement* in management, and this trend, although overlain with the effects of legalistic employee relations, continues to replace old-fashioned scientific management.

The human relations movement received a number of significant boosts during the 1930s, 1940s, and 1950s. Studies undertaken throughout mid-century showed that "When workers' hostilities, resentments, suspicions and fears were replaced by favorable attitudes, a substantial increase in production occurred."[5] Experience with the human relations approach to management has led many to conclude that:

- In most circumstances, people-centered management is more effective in inspiring productivity than production-centered management
- Closer supervision is more associated with lower productivity when compared with more general supervision.

WHERE WE ARE, WHERE WE ARE HEADING

Employees in the American work force have changed dramatically over the years. More and more workers know about their rights under today's laws or are at least aware that they have certain rights. Employees' knowledge and the stance they and their representatives (such as labor unions and external advocacy agencies) have adopted have in many instances forced management into a legalistic posture.

Authoritarianism remains with us, but it is steadily diminishing in its incidence and is probably less significant in health care than in certain other settings. Legalism remains fairly strong and is to be found in abundance in many modern organizations, health care and otherwise, as many managers deal with employees in a particular manner primarily because the law says they must. However, legalism is slowly but steadily diminishing as the humanistic philosophy of employee relations grows in acceptance. Many people are slow to adjust when faced with societal change, and although a law can force behavioral change, a law in and of itself cannot change attitudes and beliefs. The legislators who frame our laws are undoubtedly aware that much early compliance comes primarily as a result of obedience to the law, not because people wish to change their ways, but they also know that acceptance grows over time and that those people who were simply obeying the law will eventually behave as they do because to them it has become the right way.

There have always been some humanistic managers, but their considerate and people-focused style has likely arisen more from their nature as individuals than from any conscious belief in humanistic management.

Upon casual observation the legalistic and humanistic stages of employee relations may appear to be very much the same. Often the difference between the two is management's motivation: In the legalistic stage, managers provide fair and humane treatment because it is required by law and they wish to keep themselves and the organization out of legal trouble. In the humanistic stage, managers provide fair and humane treatment because they believe that doing so is the proper way to manage.

Discussion Points

1. Cite two or three commonly observable practices in present-day organizational management that indicate the presence of residual authoritarianism.
2. Identify and describe the fundamental difference between legalistic management and humanistic management, and describe some indicators that might help distinguish one from the other.
3. Present three or four reasons why authoritarian management still prevails to a considerable extent in many organizations.
4. Discuss what you believe is the primary reason why authoritarian management has prevailed for so long a time and in some places remains as solidly entrenched as ever.
5. If so-called "scientific management" was in fact the "diabolical scheme" that some considered it to be, discuss what advantages could possibly have prompted its relatively widespread adoption in the early part of the twentieth century.
6. Reduce the parallel discussion of the "job organization system" and the "cooperative motivation system" to a single

statement that reflects the greatest single difference between
the two systems.

7. Name at least three major pieces of legislation that supported
the advancement of the "human relations movement" in
management, and state how they did so.

8. Identify the primary force in moving organizational management from legalism to humanism in the years to come.

9. Explain, in terms related to employment and work, the implications of Douglas McGregor's statement: "Man lives by
bread alone, when there is no bread." How does this relate
to employee motivation?

10. Identify one organizational setting—look outside of health
care—in which strict authoritarian management is not only
prevalent but preferred. Why is this so?

NOTES

[1] Lyndall F. Urwick, "The Development of Industrial Engineering," *Industrial Engineering Handbook, Second Edition,* H. B. Maynard, Editor-in-Chief (New York: McGraw-Hill Book Company, 1963), Section 1, p. 5.

[2] Rensis Likert, *New Patterns of Management* (New York: McGraw-Hill Book Company, 1961).

[3] Douglas M. McGregor, "The Human Side of Enterprise," *Management Review,* Vol. 46, No. 11 (November 1957), pp. 22-28.

[4] A. H. Maslow, "A Theory of Human Motivation," *Psychological Review,* Vol. 50, 1943, pp. 370-396.

[5] Rensis Likert, "Motivation and Increased Productivity," *Management Record,* Vol. 18, No. 4 (April 1956), pp. 128-131.

CHAPTER 9

The Health Care Manager and Employee Problems

This chapter—

- Concedes the inevitability of people problems in any work group and explores the more likely origins of such problems
- Establishes the primary purpose of most processes for dealing with employee problems as correction of behavior
- Differentiates between problems of performance and problems of behavior, and presents systematic processes for addressing each
- Offers guidance for addressing employee absenteeism
- Describes the applicability and operation of an employee assistance program
- Differentiates between common forms of termination for cause (behavior problems and performance problems)
- Stresses the need to emphasize problem prevention whenever possible
- Highlights factors that affect a department manager's ability to take corrective action when needed
- Emphasizes the need to document employee performance and behavior problems.

THE INEVITABILITY OF PEOPLE PROBLEMS

A chronic personnel problem involving differences between some staff members of two adjoining hospital departments had surfaced once again, this time resulting in a meeting involving two department managers, several rank-and-file employees, and an employee relations manager. After more than an hour of animated discussion during which charges and counter-charges flew, the employees were excused and the others continued for another half-hour. When the meeting finally broke up, some 90 minutes had gone by and only the most tentative of conclusions had been reached. As the participants rose to leave the room, the pager worn by one of the department managers sounded.

The manager checked the pager's message and muttered, "I was expecting this. Looks like another of my pet troublemakers is acting up again." On the way out of the room this manager also remarked in a voice strained with frustration, "You know, I could probably get some *real* work done around here if it weren't for all these people problems that keep popping up."

We perhaps have to sympathize with the frustrated manager to some extent; most managers have more than enough to do without spending inordinate amounts of their time "baby-sitting" adults. However, the manager who feels frustration because of people problems needs to appreciate that, like it or not, people problems are part of the legitimate terrain of the first-line manager. The first-line manager, the person who supervises the people who perform the hands-on work, is to a considerable extent a frustration fighter by definition. People problems are a legitimate part of this person's role in maintaining rank-and-file employees as effective producers, and if there were substantially fewer people problems occurring, chances are that correspondingly fewer first-line managers would be needed in our work organizations.

As long as there are people in the workplace, we can expect people problems. Problems with staff will never completely disappear, except perhaps for a few functions that may be taken over by automated equipment, and then we can probably expect mechanical problems to replace people problems.

Although for many people it may be one of the less appealing aspects of being a manager, dealing with people problems is an inevitable and unavoidable part of the department manager's role.

Sources of People Problems

Problems presented by employees can arise because of job-related difficulties, personal problems experienced largely outside of work, or a combination of the two. Regarding personal problems, some people are much better than others at keeping the working side and the personal side of their lives separate from each other, but it is not possible to completely separate the person on the job from the person off the job. Problems flow both ways; personal problems come to work and often affect job performance and relationships, and work-related problems go home and often affect one's personal life and relationships.

One could certainly say that an employee's personal problems are no business of the manager, and be correct—up to a point. If an individual's personal problems are manifesting themselves in deteriorating performance, reduced productivity, or disruption of the department's ability to function normally, the manager must become interested because of these negative effects on operations.

When an employee who has performed satisfactorily for a prolonged period and has always gotten along with others reasonably well begins to shows signs of performance and relationship problems on the job, the manager has every reason to suspect that there is some underlying problem behind this changed behavior. It may not be evident initially whether the problem has its basis in the workplace or on the outside, but the results of the changed behavior—the emerging performance or relationship problems—are the manager's immediate concern.

The Manager's Response

Should you suspect that a personal problem is behind an individual's decline in performance, you must approach the employee in a manner that is respectful of his or her right to privacy. Although the performance resulting from an individual's behavior must be addressed for the sake of the department and the people served, what may be occurring in the individual's private life is no business of yours.

Accordingly, always address the results of behavior; never attempt to infer causes. Tell the individual what is being done wrong and how it should be done right, and provide whatever help the person needs to take appropriate corrective action. Do not under any circumstances probe for personal information. Make it plain that you are there to listen if the person wants to talk, but do not ask the individual what is wrong if the problem seems to lie outside of the work situation.

Should an employee volunteer information concerning personal problems, listen and prepare to refer the employee elsewhere as necessary. Even if an employee reveals his or her problem and asks you for advice, do not respond as requested. You may feel flattered that the employee thinks enough of you to reveal a personal problem and ask for your advice, but unless you are a professional working in one of the human services areas it is best to keep your advice to yourself.

Some of the most troublesome statements a manager can make under the circumstances start with "If I were you. . . ."

Refer the troubled employee to the appropriate point from which he or she may be directed toward the proper source of knowledgeable help. Usually this will mean referral to the employee health service or the organization's employee assistance program (EAP).

PRIMARY PURPOSE: CORRECTION

Throughout this chapter we will make a number of references to *corrective* processes. Although there will be instances in which the action taken concerning an employee problem is undeniably and unavoidably punitive in character, the primary purpose of action taken concerning employee performance or behavior should be correction of that behavior. We will of course speak of disciplinary action. *Disciplinary* is the nature of action that addresses *discipline*, and a quick check in the dictionary shows that one prominent definition of discipline is *teaching, especially to correct*. Discipline in turn has its roots in the word *disciple*, which is a *learner, pupil,* or *follower*.

Correction is always the primary intent of what we refer to as corrective processes. The primary objective of disciplinary action should also always be correction of behavior. Yet there is a seemingly unavoidable punitive dimension to most ways of addressing rule breaking or policy violation, since so much management response to these kinds of behavior involves "warnings." Even though we accept the sometimes-punitive aspect of true disciplinary action, we do not want to see an employee with a performance problem treated in a punitive manner. Therefore, it should be considered essential to separate problems of performance from true behavior problems.

SEPARATE ISSUES OF PERFORMANCE AND BEHAVIOR

The department manager will find it necessary to address different kinds of problems presented by employees on the job, specifically problems of performance and problems of behavior. Most of the time these kinds of problems must be addressed using different approaches:

Performance problems are problems meeting the expectations or requirements of the job and problems doing the work and producing the minimum level of quality or output required. Performance problems are not the same as behavior problems, and they should not be addressed in the same manner.

Behavior problems are those that involve violations of policies or work rules. These are problems of conduct. Most of the time they may be considered completely unrelated to performance and may have no bearing whatsoever on how the employee is performing on the job.

It is sometimes necessary to try to determine whether a particular employee *cannot* perform as expected, calling for the manager to address a performance problem, or *will not* perform as expected, perhaps requiring disciplinary action. This area of overlap occurs occasionally when an individual's deliberate acts or acts of recklessness, negligence, or carelessness bring about deterioration of performance to below accepted standards. In other words, when one *cannot* perform it is a performance problem; when one *will not* perform it is a behavior problem.

Thorough orientation and education are necessary for all employees. Employees are always entitled to know what is expected of them, whether related to performance or behavior. Concerning behavior, it is essential that the employee know all the applicable policies and work rules. Concerning performance, it is essential that the employee has been trained thoroughly and given every opportunity (consistent with what others have been given) to learn the job.

Whether behavior or performance seems to be involved, the department manager should first examine what was expected of the employee: Was this person fully knowledgeable of the expected behavior or performance?

Addressing Performance Problems

When an employee appears to be falling short of expected performance, perhaps falling behind in output, turning out poor quality, or simply doing things incorrectly, as department manager the first place to look for the source of the problem is yourself (or perhaps your immediate predecessor, if you have been in place only a short while). The critical question to ask is: Did I (or my predecessor) do everything reasonably possible to help this employee succeed?

Performance problems, especially those occurring fairly early in a person's employment, are often the result of weak or sketchy orientation. To address a performance problem the department manager must positively identify the problem and proceed to work out, preferably with the participation of the employee, what must be done to correct the difficulty and by when it must be done. The performance improvement process might proceed in the following manner:

- The manager observes a problem situation involving substandard performance in some form (e.g., unacceptable quality, insufficient productivity, complaints of patients, visitors, or others).
- The manager investigates to verify the problem, making sure of the facts before addressing the situation with the employee as performance needing correction.
- The manager meets privately with the employee to point out, discuss, and elicit the employee's perspective on the perceived difficulty. (For more about one-on-one meetings of this kind, refer to the section on counseling in Chapter 11, Addressing Problems before Corrective Action).
- The manager should make every reasonable effort to secure the employee's agreement concerning the nature of the problem and what needs to be done to correct the unacceptable performance. Ideally the two should agree on a brief written description of what is wrong and what is needed for correction.
- This agreement should include a timetable for correction, with the two parties agreeing on when corrective action must be accomplished. Part of this agreement should specify whether there will be interim checkpoints at which to examine progress. (If complete correction requires 90 days, for example, the manager might schedule meetings to evaluate progress at 30 and 60 days.)
- At whatever evaluate points are established, it is critical that the manager follow up thoroughly and on time.
- At the end of the evaluation period the manager has to decide whether the employee's performance has improved as required, improved only partly, not improved, or perhaps deteriorated even further.

The desired result of this process is of course the employee's return to acceptable performance. Depending on the results, however, other possible subsequent steps are: (1) extending the improvement period (in the case of partial improvement) or (2) dismissing the employee for failure to meet job standards.

What about the employee who corrects his or her performance well enough to get by the correction period, and then goes back to substandard performance some weeks or months later? The department manager may elect to go through the performance improvement process with this employee again but will probably not be willing to do so a third time. Whatever documentation is created the second time through, the process should include wording to the effect that this time performance must remain at or above standard or the person's employment is at risk.

Exhibit 9-1 presents a model procedure for addressing the need for improvement in performance.

Exhibit 9-1   Model Policy and Procedure: Performance Improvement Process

The following procedure is provided to establish clear direction for the resolution of problems concerning an employee's substandard job performance.

Substandard performance is defined as: A demonstrated lack of acceptable work performance, or chronically unsatisfactory results that prevent an employee from attaining or maintaining job standard.

Job standard is defined as: The average or acceptable level of output provided by employees in the same or similar position or classification, or the standard level of results defined in advance by the department manager clearly identifying the quality or quantity of output expected.

In the event that a non-probationary employee exhibits substandard performance of job duties or fails to fulfill all the responsibilities of his or her position, the department manager should initially make a sincere and adequate effort to guide the employee in returning to standard performance by:

- Verifying the job standard for accuracy and applicability, and making any necessary adjustments
- Advising and guiding the employee in the creation of a plan for the employee's return to standard performance and a time frame for doing so, documenting this effort using a Counseling form (Attachment A)
- Guiding and monitoring the employee's efforts to attain standard performance
- Removing obstacles to the employee's progress where possible.

In the event that the employee does not attain job standard within the agreed-upon time, the department manager should next:

- Complete a Work Improvement Evaluation (Attachment B)
- Repeat the creation of a mutually agreed upon plan of action, this time including referral to Employee Relations or Employee

---

continues

Exhibit 9-1   Model Policy and Procedure: Performance Improvement Process (continued)

Health if applicable (should there be some indication of underlying difficulty).

If this second effort is unsuccessful in returning the employee to standard performance within the agreed-upon time:

- Complete a Performance Expectations form (Attachment C) placing the employee on notice of probationary status and calling for dismissal for substandard performance no later than 30 days following this final notice unless standard performance is attained during that period.

Note: Once an employee has been through the Performance Expectations stage and has again achieved standard performance, that person's performance is expected to remain at standard or better indefinitely. Absent extenuating circumstances (for example, undergoing a corrective or rehabilitative process under an Employee Assistance Program or the auspices of Employee Health), reversion to substandard performance will result in dismissal.

Exhibit 9-1, Attachment A

Counseling Form

= Performance Counseling

= Probationary Counseling

= Other _____

Employee Name: _____ ID No. _____

Department: _____ Hire Date _____

Job Title/Grade _____ Job Date _____

Summary of discussion:

Action to be taken by manager:

Action to be taken by employee:

continues

Exhibit 9-1   Model Policy and Procedure: Performance Improvement Process (continued)

Date of Follow-Up Meeting: _____

Employee Signature: _____ Date: _____

Manager Signature: _____ Date: _____

Exhibit 9-1, Attachment B

Work Improvement Evaluation

This document summarizes a work improvement discussion between the manager and the employee. An initial effort to correct a documented performance problem was unsuccessful, indicating the need for additional corrective action represented by the numbered objectives below that must be met to return the employee to an acceptable level of performance.

No.   Description of objective and the agreed-upon plan for achievement

1.

2.

3.

Referral to Employee Relations or Employee Health as appropriate: _____

Date of next review: _____

Signatures:

Employee _____

Manager _____

Date Discussed _____

continues

Exhibit 9-1   Model Policy and Procedure: Performance Improvement Process (continued)

Exhibit 9-1, Attachment C

Performance Expectations

Employee Name: _____ ID No. _____

Department: _____ Hire Date _____

Job Title/Grade _____ Job Date _____

Summary of performance-problem discussion:

Follow-up was performed on the following dates:

_____   _____

_____   _____

Continued substandard performance makes it necessary to place the employee on a probationary status subject to dismissal during or after 30 days from the date of signing unless fully satisfactory and lasting improvement is demonstrated by the employee.

Employee Signature: _____ Date: _____

Manager Signature: _____ Date: _____

Addressing Behavior Problems

Several courses of action are available for addressing behavior problems.

Disciplinary Action

"A chief reason why supervisors don't confront problem employee behavior is that they are uncomfortable with the traditional punitive discipline systems many have to use."[1] This quotation says a great deal about why supervisors frequently shy away from disciplinary action even when it may be deserved. The systems they use may or may not be overly punitive in how they operate, but the majority of employees (and their supervisors and managers as well) will likely *perceive* their disciplinary systems as punitive. And few managers look forward to delivering disciplinary action.

Although we cannot help but regard the majority of disciplinary actions as punitive to some extent, in all but certain severe instances that involve immediate termination, the purpose of disciplinary action remains the correction of behavior.

The mere thought of having to take disciplinary action is without a doubt upsetting and unsettling to many managers. Impending disciplinary action makes the manager apprehensive, and the manager will sometimes react in a manner that is not much healthier than the misconduct it is supposed to be addressing. Some managers will simply back away from the situation, postponing action until they can allow themselves to forget it entirely. Others will approach disciplinary action hesitantly and timidly, watering it down to such an extent that it becomes ineffective.

However, disciplinary action is much like any number of other difficult tasks that fall to the manager in that conscientious attention to the process, plus practice in applying it, eventually lead to a degree of familiarity that will allow the manager to apply disciplinary action honestly and confidently when needed. It is doubtful that most managers ever become entirely comfortable with the process, and we might go so far as to suggest that one should never become "comfortable" in applying a process that can conceivably affect employment and even careers.

The Progressive Discipline Process
The complete progressive disciplinary process consists of:

- Counseling
- Oral warning
- Written warning
- Suspension
- Termination.

Certain lesser violations, such as absenteeism or chronic tardiness, may go through all of the steps beginning with counseling, progressing through oral warning and written warning for repeat violations, and ultimately through suspension without pay and eventually to termination if correction cannot be effected. With such supposedly minor infractions it may even be advisable to repeat a step or drop back a step in the progression if there has been a significant time lapse between infractions.

Disciplinary action cannot always be progressive, however. Some infractions may involve two steps only. For example, sleeping on the job might call for a written warning for the initial offense and termination for a second offense.

Some infractions, usually clearly spelled out in policy manuals and employee handbooks, call for immediate termination (although often following suspension pending investigation as necessary). These one-strike-and-out transgressions ordinarily include the likes of fighting or physical assault, using illegal drugs or alcohol on the job, carrying a weapon on the premises, and theft. (One might be quick to point out that immediate termination with no change to one's behavior is hardly "corrective"; then again, we might reason that when an employee is released for a serious infraction we have corrected the *problem* by removing its cause.)

Exhibit 9-2 presents a sample progressive discipline policy and procedure, including the recommended treatment of various forms of infraction.

Exhibit 9-2   Model Policy and Procedure: Progressive Discipline

The Hospital is committed to providing the best possible working conditions for all employees. Rules of conduct have been established to assist the Hospital and its employees in achieving the goals of the organization as well as providing a safe and productive work environment. Each employee is expected to observe all rules of conduct and to follow the instructions provided by his or her immediate supervisor. Supervisors and managers are responsible for applying the rules to all employees fairly and consistently.

When an employee appears to have violated a Hospital rule, the immediate supervisor should address the specific problem through the progressive discipline process.

A.   **Steps in Progressive Discipline**
1. Counseling
   Before informal or formal disciplinary action it is the supervisor's responsibility to counsel the employee to correct the undesirable

continues

Exhibit 9-2 Model Policy and Procedure: Progressive Discipline (continued)

behavior. Utilize the Counseling Form (Exhibit 9-1, Attachment A), which is then retained in departmental files unless the employee is eventually terminated, at which time the form is forwarded to Human Resources.

2. **Oral Warning**

   a. An informal disciplinary conference may be scheduled when an employee repeatedly displays undesirable behavior and does not respond to counseling. The conference should be recorded on the Record of Oral Warning (Attachment A), which is retained in the department manager's files.

   b. If further disciplinary action is necessary for the same offense, the Record of Oral Warning should be forwarded to Human Resources for inclusion in the employee's personnel file.

3. **Written Warning**

   a. If counselings and oral warnings fail to correct the employee's behavior, a Written Warning should be generated. The employee will be informed that the Record of Oral Warning and the Written Warning will be included in the personnel file, he or she will be ineligible for transfer for six (6) months, and repetition of the offense will lead to serious disciplinary action such as suspension without pay or termination of employment.

   b. An employee whose inappropriate behavior has not been corrected by counseling, oral warning, or written warning will be referred to Employee Relations for further counseling or to Employee Health or Employee Assistance for evaluation and referrals if appropriate.

4. **Suspension Without Pay**

   a. A temporary termination of work at the will of the employer may be initiated if the employee fails to respond to the foregoing steps. Time off may be waived at the discretion of the manager if staffing needs require the employee's presence, but waiver of time off does not lessen the severity of the disciplinary action.

   b. At the discretion of the manager, indefinite suspension pending investigation may be utilized to provide time and opportunity to thoroughly investigate an alleged violation that has the potential to result in termination.

5. **Discharge**

   Termination of employment for violation of Hospital rules may apply after repeated counseling, warnings, referrals, and suspensions or after initial commission of specific severe violations.

continues

Exhibit 9-2   Model Policy and Procedure: Progressive Discipline (continued)

6. General

The Hospital reserves the right to amend its rules as necessary. Each manager has the right to initiate the progressive disciplinary process at any step, depending on the seriousness of the offense. It is required that all violations leading to potential suspension without pay or discharge be reviewed with Human Resources.

B. Violations and Severity

1. *Carelessness:* Careless acts that could result in personal injury to patients, employees or visitors, or damage to property.
   a. First violation: Written warning.
   b. Second violation: Up to 5-day suspension without pay.
   c. Third violation: Discharge.
2. *Insubordination:* An employee's refusal to comply with a reasonable and safe work instruction as required by the immediate supervisor.
   a. First violation: Up to 5-day suspension without pay, and Employee Relations referral.
   b. Second violation: Discharge.
3. *Absenteeism: Excessive* absenteeism is the frequent use of sick time which in the judgment of the department manager adversely affects the operation of the department, regularly occurs before or after scheduled days off, weekends, holidays, or scheduled vacations, or results in sick time being used as it accrues. *Unexcused* absenteeism is absence without timely notice to the manager or designee prior to the start of the scheduled shift, per departmental policy.
   a. First violation: Oral warning.
   b. Second violation: Written warning and referral to Employee Health for counseling.
   c. Third violation: Up to three-day suspension without pay.
   d. Fourth violation: Discharge.
   Note: Failure to appear at work or call in per policy for three consecutive work days will result in discharge for job abandonment.
4. *Tardiness:* Consistent tardiness is the patterned failure to report for work at the designated starting time.
   a. First violation: Oral warning.
   b. Second violation: Written warning and referral to Employee Relations for counseling.
   c. Third violation: Up to three-day suspension without pay.
   d. Fourth violation: Discharge.

continues

**Exhibit 9-2   Model Policy and Procedure: Progressive
Discipline** (continued)

5. *Misconduct:* Actions detrimental to the interests of the Hospital or which cause harm or disruption to any person or Hospital activity. Some examples are: threatening or discourteous behavior toward patients or visitors; sexual harassment; misuse of confidential information; leaving the work area without permission; gambling; possession of explosives, firearms or other weapons on Hospital property, violation of safe practices in the performance of work.

   a. First violation: Written warning and up to five-day suspension without pay, plus referral to Employee Relations for Counseling.

   b. Second violation: Discharge.

6. *Sleeping:* Sleeping on the job is prohibited unless it is recognized as a legitimate part of an employee's extended shift.

   a. First violation: Written warning and up to five-day suspension without pay, plus referral to Employee Relations or Employee Health for Counseling.

   b. Second violation: Discharge.

7. *Solicitation:* Employees may not engage in unauthorized solicitation, distribution, or posting of materials on Hospital premises.

   a. First violation: Written warning.

   b. Second violation: Written warning and up to three-day suspension without pay.

   c. Third violation: Discharge.

8. *Falsification of Information:* Falsification of information on employment applications or in other work situations is prohibited. This prohibition includes the making of false entries on time records or punching another employee's time card.

   a. First violation: Indefinite suspension pending investigation prior to possible discharge.

9. *Alcohol and Illegal Drugs:* Possession or use of being under the influence of alcohol or illegal drugs on Hospital premises is prohibited. Employees using prescription medications while at work are requested to report such use to the appropriate manager.

   Because of the considerable responsibility that all employees have for the Hospital's patients, the manager who has probable cause to believe an employee to be under the influence of alcohol or drugs may ask the employee to voluntarily submit to an appropriate test arranged by either Employee Health or the Emergency Department. Refusal to submit to such reasonable request may result in disciplinary action.

   a. First violation: Indefinite suspension pending test results and, if necessary, the employee's willingness to enter an approved

continues

Exhibit 9-2   Model Policy and Procedure: Progressive Discipline (continued)

rehabilitation program as determined by the employee's personal physician and Employee Health.

b. Second violation: Discharge.

10. *Unauthorized Possession of Property.* The unauthorized use, possession, or removal of Hospital property or the property of patients, visitors, employees, or others.

a. First violation: Indefinite suspension pending investigation prior to possible discharge.

Exhibit 9-2, Attachment A

Record of Oral Warning

Employee Name: _____ ID No. _____

Department: _____ Hire Date _____

Job Title/Grade _____ Job Date _____

Specific problem or incident, and rule or policy reviewed and discussed:

Dates of previous discussions or counselings relating to the foregoing:

Action required of employee:

Employee Signature: _____ Date: _____

Manager Signature: _____ Date: _____

This record will be maintained in departmental files. If further action is required for the same offense, it will be forwarded to Human Resources for inclusion in the personnel file.

continues

Exhibit 9-2 Model Policy and Procedure: Progressive Discipline (continued)

Exhibit 9-2, Attachment B

Written Warning

Employee Name: _____ ID No. _____

Department: _____ Hire Date _____

Job Title/Grade _____ Job Date _____

Specific problem or incident, and rule or policy reviewed and discussed:

Dates of previous discussions, counselings, or warnings relating to the foregoing:

Action required of employee:

Employee Signature: _____ Date: _____

Manager Signature: _____ Date: _____

This record puts the employee on notice that additional violations will result in more serious disciplinary action such as suspension without pay or discharge.

Exhibit 9-2, Attachment C

Suspension Without Pay

Employee Name: _____ ID No. _____

Department: _____ Hire Date _____

Job Title/Grade _____ Job Date _____

continues

Exhibit 9-2   Model Policy and Procedure: Progressive Discipline (continued)

Specific problem or incident, and rule or policy reviewed and discussed:

Previous actions taken:

Date   **Action Taken**

Suspended for _____ days from above date;
report back on _____
_____Time off waived by manager for the following reason
(waiver does not lessen the severity of the action).

Employee Signature: _____ Date: _____

Manager Signature: _____ Date: _____

This is a final warning. Failure to respond appropriately may result in discharge.

_____

Exhibit 9-2, Attachment D

Notice of Discharge or Dismissal

Employee Name:_____ ID No. _____

Department: _____ Hire Date _____

Job Title/Grade _____ Job Date _____

You are being terminated from employment with the Hospital for the following reasons:

continues

Exhibit 9-2   Model Policy and Procedure: Progressive Discipline (continued)

Previous actions taken:

Date   **Action Taken**

_____ Check here to indicate whether the employee desires an exit interview to discuss benefit status. If the employee declines this opportunity, continuation of benefits information will be mailed to the employee's home address.

Employee Signature: _____ Date: _____

Manager Signature: _____ Date: _____

This is a final warning. Failure to respond appropriately may result in discharge.

The initial step in many instances is informal counseling. Counseling is best undertaken when the manager observes the employee headed into troublesome territory but not yet at the point of requiring disciplinary action.

The oral warning is actually the first supposedly "official" step in the progressive disciplinary process. Although it is called an oral warning and is delivered orally to the employee, the manager is always advised to make a written record of it (many organizations have forms specifically designated for documenting oral warnings) and ask the employee to review and sign it. Why can it be "oral" and still have to be written? First, although a record is made of it, in many instances this record never goes into an employee's personnel file *unless* the infraction is followed by a similar infraction requiring a written warning. Second, documentation is essential to prove, if need be, that the organization's processes were followed. If a disciplinary policy states that an oral warning will be the first level for a given infraction, it may later be necessary to prove that the oral warning was indeed given (see Chapter 12, Employee Documentation: Should and Should-Nots for the Manager).

At all steps of the disciplinary process the affected employee is asked to review and sign the documentation created. The manager may need to stress that signing does not necessarily indicate agreement with the action, but rather simply acknowledges that the employee has seen the document, has been provided with a copy, and has discussed the problem with the manager. It is not unusual, however, for an employee to refuse to sign a warning even to acknowledge its receipt. When this occurs, the manager should simply note in the signature area "Employee refused to sign" and make certain that the document is dated. In difficult circumstances in which the manager has reason to believe that the disagreement may escalate and involve others both internally and perhaps externally, it is suggested that another manager witness the employee's refusal to sign and so note on the document.

EMPLOYEE ABSENTEEISM

Some degree of absenteeism is accepted as a fact of organizational life. People become legitimately ill and experience family emergencies and other urgent matters that sometimes keep them away from work. However, as many department managers have discovered, it is not possible to clearly recognize the extremely fine line between acceptable and unacceptable levels of absenteeism.

Some department managers appear to pay little or no attention to employee absenteeism. But if the manager seems not to notice absenteeism or conveys what is essentially a "hands off" attitude toward it, chances are that absenteeism will be higher than it needs to be.

Absenteeism costs money. While someone may be receiving paid time off for being away from work, a job that must be covered—in health care, for example, a direct caregiver position—incurs the direct cost of a temporary replacement or staff overtime. For other jobs—say a support position of some kind—there may be no need for one-to-one replacement for a day or so, but the department will experience lost productivity as a result of the absence.

Experience with traditional sick-time benefits programs has suggested that an organization's sick-time benefit can breed its own usage. For example, consider the experience of two health care organizations in the same community, one providing a benefit of 12 sick days per year and the other providing 5 days per year. In the facility where employees received 12 days per year, the average usage per employee was approximately 7 days per year. In the facility where employees received 5 days per year, the average usage per employee was just slightly more than 3 days per year. One might logically conclude that the organization with the higher rate of sick-time consumption did not necessarily have unhealthier employees than the other facility.

It is such experiences with sick time that have encouraged an increasing number of organizations to reduce their absolute sick time benefit and combine it with vacation and other personal time into a paid-time-off bank. Under these kinds of plans, the person who uses little or no time off for illness has the time left for other uses.

A department manager's obvious conscientious attention to absenteeism is a significant factor in controlling absenteeism. Some employees will be inclined to abuse sick time if they see that the manager seems to pay no attention to their absences. They come to regard the lack of attention as approval of their conduct, which it in fact is if only by default.

For the control of absenteeism in the department:

- You cannot clearly remember everyone's attendance, so keep accurate attendance records. Do not depend on having to ask the payroll section to dig out a person's attendance record; keep track yourself so you are constantly in touch with attendance.
- Check in with employees after they return from an absence, even of a single day. A simple question, perhaps "Feel better today?" or "Good to have you back" lets employees know that you are aware of their attendance.
- Watch for patterns of absences, one of the most reliable signs of sick-time abuse. The most common are "holiday stretching," being absent the day before or the day after a scheduled holiday, or "weekend stretching," being absent on Friday or Monday. It has long been known that more employees tend to be "sick" on Monday than on any other day of the week.
- Counsel any employee who appears to be getting close to a level of absenteeism that can trigger disciplinary action. For example, if the policy says that five instances of unexcused absence in a 12-month period call for the start of disciplinary action, meet with the individual who has been absent four times in eight months, explain the policy, and point out where he or she is heading. Do not wait until disciplinary action is called for to speak up.

- Do not avoid taking disciplinary action for absenteeism when it is deserved.

You need not be punitive; a progressive system leaves lots of room for improvement and your intent should always be to help the employee improve.

EMPLOYEE ASSISTANCE PROGRAMS

An employee assistance program (EAP) says to employees that the organization cares about them beyond the organizational needs of the moment. An EAP provides information, assessment, advice, and referral for employees who are experiencing personal problems that can affect them as individuals and as producers. Employees who take advantage of the EAP will experience confidential assessment, which is ordinarily followed by referral to an appropriate source of professional help.

It is common practice to use an external assessment and referral source rather than have employees (for example, someone in Human Resources) perform this function. This helps preserve employee confidentiality and allows employees to build a level of confidence in the EAP. For obvious reasons, many employees are more likely to take up personal issues with a person outside of the organization.

Improvements brought about through an EAP ordinarily take some time. There may be a temptation to look for short-term improvement, however, rather than long-term benefit to both the employee and the organization.

Consideration of some of the kinds of problems addressed through an EAP suggest that "quick fixes" should not be expected:

- Substance abuse (drugs or alcohol)
- Marital or family problems
- Financial problems
- Compulsive gambling.

Most EAPs ordinarily provide for up to two or three counseling sessions to determine the appropriate referral path. After these initial visits, the individual's health insurance or other applicable program takes over.

An employee can enter an EAP through self-referral, that is, by contacting the EAP voluntarily, or the employee can be referred by management or by the employee health office. If an employee's problem can potentially negatively affect performance or present danger or risk to people or property, the organization can mandate referral to the EAP and require completion of a subsequent program (such as alcohol rehabilitation) as a condition of continued employment. The nature of the problem remains no business of the manager, but the effects on performance and on other people are indeed the manager's business.

An EAP usually costs the organization a certain nominal amount of money per employee or per full-time equivalent (FTE), often amounting to very little cost overall. Often the EAP for an entire year will cost less than the direct and indirect costs avoided through salvaging one or two employees who might otherwise have been lost.

To fully serve its intended purpose, an EAP requires:

- Top management support
- Adequate funding
- An efficient and confidential assessment and referral process
- Record-keeping that ensures confidentiality
- Manager and employee education.

An employee assistance program can sometimes relieve the department manager of an extremely difficult problem involving an ordinarily good employee who gets into trouble. The EAP can effectively assist the "nice person" for whom there would be no remaining alternative except termination if there were no EAP. And the department manager may find that there is far more satisfaction in helping salvage one employee who might otherwise fail than there is in firing countless others.

WHEN TERMINATION IS NECESSARY

The two most common kinds of involuntary employment separation are dismissal and discharge. As the terms are used here, *dismissal* relates to performance, while *discharge* relates to conduct and behavior.

Dismissal is the appropriate path for an employee who must be released due to performance problems. This will apply to the newer employee who is unable to gain sufficient control of the job to pass the probationary period, and it may apply as well to the employee who slips into performance problems and does not respond to corrective processes. Dismissal should be the final resort following all reasonable efforts to improve performance.

As terminations go, dismissal is the equivalent of layoff; it is something of a "no-fault" separation in that it concedes only that the person did not fit this particular kind of work, and it makes no judgments about the person's ability to succeed elsewhere. And as is the case with layoff, the individual separated via dismissal can be considered eligible for unemployment compensation.

Discharge, which is related to conduct and behavior, is termination for cause—what is commonly referred to as "fired." Discharge should occur only following appropriate application of the organization's progressive disciplinary process and failure to correct the offending behavior. An employee who is discharged for cause is ordinarily considered ineligible for unemployment compensation (but whether the employee receives it is not up to the organization but rather an external agency).

No employee, no matter the nature of the infraction, should ever be summarily discharged, that is, fired on the spot or, especially, fired in anger. The appropriate reaction to even the most blatant of one-strike-and-gone offenses is to immediately place the person on indefinite suspension pending discharge. This provides a cooling-off period for all concerned, and it provides time for a fair and thorough investigation as needed.

Dismissal and discharge are addressed in more detail in Chapter 13, Terminating Employees: Minimizing the Legal Risks.

PARTNERSHIP WITH HUMAN RESOURCES

Disciplinary action is one area in which the department manager and Human Resources frequently collide. Conflicts can be minimized, however, by having clearly stated policies governing who is responsible for what parts of the process. A significant number of organizations require managers to coordinate all disciplinary actions with Human Resources. This is a reasonable requirement: Human Resources can help provide consistency and ensure that all legalities are observed.

Human Resources should be allowed to serve as a central monitor of disciplinary actions, initially rendering an opinion as to whether a proposed action is appropriate to the situation. Another important aspect of the HR role in discharge is to ensure that all of the proper steps called for in the organization's policy have been applied.

PREVENTION WHEN POSSIBLE

Active prevention is important in reducing disciplinary actions and keeping them to a minimum. Two keys to prevention are information and education.

Be certain that each new employee is familiar with the work rules and applicable policies, all of which should be included in the employee handbook. These may have been covered during the organization's general new-employee orientation, but do not assume so. It is essential to have them in writing.

Make sure that each new employee goes through the employee handbook and signs and turns in the handbook receipt as required. One may not necessarily be able to get an employee to read the entire handbook, but the manager can at least remind all new employees that they will be considered knowledgeable of the rules once they have turned in the signed handbook receipt.

Periodically review various rules and policies with the entire staff, perhaps covering an item or two at each routine staff meeting. Personnel policies are regularly revised and updated, and the occasion of revision presents a good reason for the review. It will be more difficult for employees to ignore the rules and policies if they are reviewed periodically.

Also important in preventing disciplinary actions is "preventive employee relations." Remain alert to signs and signals indicating that events may be heading in an inappropriate direction. If something strikes you as not quite right, talk with employees about it—do not allow it to grow into something that leads to trouble among staff and becomes more difficult to manage.

Remaining visible and available to employees (see Chapter 5, The Manager-Employee Relationship) can help prevent the need for disciplinary actions. When the department manager is available and accessible, many issues that might otherwise escalate into behavioral problems can be caught and addressed early. Also, the mere presence of the manager tends to have a stabilizing effect on the work group. Staying in touch with employees and maintaining a solid one-to-one relationship with each one will go a long way in helping prevent disciplinary problems.

FOR EFFECTIVE CORRECTIVE ACTION

Several factors affect a department manager's ability to take corrective action when needed:

- *Knowledge.* Know your organization's policies and work rules well enough that you do not have to look in a book whenever a question or problem arises. Likewise, know the progressive disciplinary process and know with whom in Human Resources you need to coordinate disciplinary actions. Take advantage of whatever training in these processes the organization offers.

- *Timing.* Do not delay deserved criticism or disciplinary action any longer than absolutely necessary. Delay only weakens the impact of the action taken and lessens its importance. The more immediate the action is, the more effective it is likely to be.
- *Consistency.* Strive for consistent treatment of employees. Work rules and policies must be applied consistently regardless of who is involved in any particular problem or infraction. This can be difficult to accomplish in instances in which some seem to be more deserving of kinder treatment than others; for example, consider two cases of chronic absenteeism, one involving an employee who you know to have chronic health problems and the other involving what is clearly sick-time abuse. As difficult as it may be to make yourself do so, employees must be dealt with equally for similar infractions.
- *Intimidation.* Do not allow yourself to be intimidated by the occasional employee who seems to be trying to exercise the upper hand in your relationship. One may be tempted to go easier on such an employee who possesses needed skills that happen to be short on the market; surely you have no desire to drive away a much-needed person. However, no employee, no matter how specialized or how valuable, can be permitted to push the boundaries of acceptable behavior and act out simply because he or she feels indispensable. Again, what applies to one must apply to all; the department cannot maintain a double standard of employee conduct. Again, the issue of consistency is probably the most important single factor in the department manager's application of corrective processes.

DOCUMENT, DOCUMENT

Most Human Resources practitioners can tell a story or two that sounds very much like this: A department manager comes to Human Resources prepared to discharge a particular employee. The HR representative hears a ringing indictment of this employee—never cooperative, the department's worst performer, the department's worst attendance record, mouthy and insubordinate and forever making trouble with other employees, and has now messed up big-time—again. The manager states "I want this person discharged—*now*." The HR person pulls the employee's personnel file and goes through it item by item. The HR representative finds no warnings, no indications of any disciplinary actions, no discussions about performance or behavior issues—nothing except several years' worth of satisfactory performance appraisals. End of discussion. Without supporting documentation of similar past difficulties, those past problems might just as well never have occurred.

This story offers a couple of lessons. First, instances in which an employee deserves some form of reprimand or formal disciplinary action should not be allowed to slide by unaddressed. Second, every such instance of reprimand or disciplinary action must be properly documented and submitted to the employee's personnel file. If there is nothing in the file about a particular problem, then for all practical purposes it never happened. (A third lesson concerns what may have been less-than-honest performance appraisals; this will be addressed in Chapter 10, Performance Appraisal: The Never-Ending Task).

Never attempt to proceed with a personnel action without generating the appropriate documentation, and always remain aware that any employee-related document you generate could conceivably go public should the employee become involved in a legal proceeding against the organization.

Discussion Points

1. Comment on the claim that "like it or not, people problems are the legitimate terrain of the first-line manager." Why is this often true to a considerable extent?
2. Explain why no employee, regardless of the apparent severity of infraction, be summarily discharged but rather be placed on indefinite suspension pending investigation.
3. Discuss why we stress that an employee's personal problems are no business of the manager. When and to what extent can the department manager be concerned with any facet of an employee's personal problem?
4. We repeatedly stress that the primary purpose of disciplinary action is *correction of behavior*. If this is indeed so, discuss why we enumerate specific behavioral problems that call for loss of employment upon a single occurrence.
5. Explain why corrective action should be taken as soon as practical following the particular infraction.

6. Explain why it is strongly recommended that problems of performance be considered separately from problems of conduct or behavior.

7. Explain why it is necessary to have a completely documented history leading up to an employee's involuntary termination, and what this documented history must be in agreement with.

8. Describe why the department manager's timely follow-up is so important in the performance improvement process.

9. Explain why is it frequently a requirement of executive management that no significant disciplinary action be implemented without the involvement of the Human Resources Department.

10. Describe the approach you might take with an employee you perceive to be "playing the gray area" with one of the so-called "lesser" infractions (for example, tardiness or attendance), repeatedly coming close to termination but cleaning up just enough to get by.

11. Explain why it would be inadvisable to skip steps in the disciplinary process leading up to an employee's involuntary termination.

12. Explain why it is considered necessary to create and retain a written record of a so-called "oral" warning?

13. Explain in detail how you would recommend addressing the problem presented by a pleasant, likeable employee whose normally marginal performance repeatedly becomes substandard a few weeks after corrective action is applied.

14. Describe two hypothetical situations in which it can be appropriate for a department manager to direct an employee into the employee assistance program (EAP) as a condition of continued employment.

15. Identify the first place a department manager should be looking for clues to corrective action when an employee exhibits problems in meeting the job's minimum standards of performance.

NOTES

[1] Jonathan A. Segal, "Did the Marquis de Sade Design Your Discipline Program?" *HR Magazine*, Vol. 35, No.9, September 1990, pp. 90-95.

CHAPTER 10

Performance Appraisal: The Never-Ending Task

This chapter—

- Highlights the principal reasons for the regular use of an up-to-date performance appraisal process
- Establishes the primary objectives of performance appraisal
- Briefly reviews a number of traditional approaches to performance appraisal
- Reviews the common obstacles to performance appraisal
- Addresses the problems presented by appraisal instruments that call for the evaluator to render personality judgments
- Establishes a sound job description as the essential starting point for an effective appraisal process
- Discusses the kinds of standards and measurements that can be applied in appraising performance
- Defines the critical difference between the terms "standard" and "average" as they are used in performance appraisal
- Discusses the two most common approaches to appraisal timing
- Describes the scheduling and conduct of the essential performance appraisal interview
- Describes when and how self-appraisal can be a constructive element of the performance appraisal process
- Briefly discusses the features of the most practical performance appraisal forms
- Reviews the important legal implications of performance appraisal
- Details the role of Human Resources in performance appraisal, indicating those points in the process at which the department manager becomes involved.

PERFORMANCE APPRAISAL: WHAT, WHY, AND HOW

The "what," "why," and "how" of performance appraisal demonstrate its key role establishing and maintaining employee performance.

What

Performance appraisal is the periodic examination of employee performance to ascertain how well the employee is performing relative to what is expected, usually accompanied by the creation of a permanent record for the employee's personnel file.

Different organizations may apply different names to the process. The more common are performance evaluation, performance review, and performance assessment. A newer term that has crept into the language of management in some places is "performance management." Some of its proponents would have us believe that performance management is somehow different and more thorough than performance appraisal, but this appears to be something of a word game. Performance management purports to encompass not only evaluation but also the overall development and improvement of the employee as a producer, quite literally managing the employee's performance, with the implication that mere performance appraisal does not do so. However, when accomplished correctly, performance appraisal includes everything that performance management claims to include.

Why

The more prevalent uses of performance appraisal are to:

- Facilitate improvement in employee performance
- Provide formal, official feedback to employees concerning performance
- Provide information for decisions concerning compensation and other personnel transactions (promotions, transfers, etc.).

In broad terms, the primary purpose of performance appraisal is to improve performance in the employee's present job. A secondary purpose is to maintain this acceptable performance.

The developmental aspects of performance appraisal include an important two-sided objective:

- Showing the employee who seeks to advance in the organization what he or she should be doing to become prepared for greater responsibility
- Identifying for management those employees who are potentially capable of advancement.

It is also a significant objective of performance appraisal to periodically remind employees of what is expected of them. This is extremely important in management's day-to-day dealings with employees; every employee is entitled to know exactly what is expected of him or her at any time.

As viewed from the perspective of the individual employee, performance appraisal should enable the employee to judge:

- In the opinion of my immediate supervisor, how am I presently performing?
- What, if anything, must I do to improve my performance?

Another important "why" for performance appraisal in health care is that it is expected, and in fact mandated, by the requirements of the organizations and agencies that accredit and regulate health care facilities. In some instances, unfortunately, mandated appraisal has led to performance appraisal systems that are little more than a formality, steps the organization must take to satisfy bureaucratic rules and provide the correct piece of paper in the files for the various surveyors to see.

How

A variety of methods have been employed in the assessment of employee performance. Most prevalent are systems that employ *rating scales* of some kind, based on comparison of an employee's performance against some scale that represents expectations. Most of the discussion in this chapter centers on the rating-scale approach to appraisal. However, other approaches sometimes used include:

- *Essay* in which the manager, perhaps once or twice each year, describes employee performance at whatever length is considered necessary, discusses the contents with the employee, and provides a copy for the personnel file

- *Critical incident* approach in which whatever occurs outside of the ordinary (positive or negative) is written up and retained for the annual or semiannual performance discussion
- *Employee comparison*, in which the employees in a group are compared with each other and ranked in order from "best" performer to "poorest" performer, or in which employees are fitted into a predetermined pattern that assumes there will be, for example, a certain percentage above average, a certain percentage below average, and the remainder in a band between
- *Checklist* approaches in which the evaluating manager must, for each evaluation criterion, describe employee performance by choosing from among a number of prepared statements (for example, the evaluator must indicate which of five statements about quality of work best describes and which least describes the employee)
- Participative approaches such as *management by objectives* (MBO), most applicable to higher-level technical and professional employees and managers.

Under certain circumstances each of these has been used to reasonable effect. Although every appraisal system has shortcomings, a rating-scale approach of the kind described in this chapter is probably the most useful and the most equitable when it is applied correctly.

Enough has been learned about performance and its appraisal to state that it is neither appropriate nor fair to base appraisal on the comparison of one person's performance against another's. Rather, accumulated experience with appraisal systems suggests that the most useful comparison that can be made via appraisal is the comparison of an employee's performance with his or her performance over time, from one evaluation period to the next.

Regardless of the specifics of a given appraisal system, it is essential that evaluators and employees have similar expectations of how their organization's system works.

NOT EVERY MANAGER'S FAVORITE TASK

Appraisal occurs sufficiently seldom that it is sometimes difficult to consider performance appraisal as a regular part of the manager's job. Therefore, when appraisal time comes around the manager may tend to view the process as extraneous and intrusive. Add to this view of appraisal as "extra work" the natural reluctance many have to address certain kinds of issues, especially those requiring criticism of others, and we can perhaps understand why appraisal is so often dreaded or disliked.

Many managers are uneasy about criticizing employees, especially in a performance appraisal situation that results in a permanent record in an employee's file and that could also affect the person's pay, job future, and perhaps even career.

One extremely common way of dealing with evaluation anxiety or fear is to ignore the appraisal requirement or to avoid it for as long as possible, then simply gloss over the task in no-fault fashion simply to have the paper to show for it. However, in business, and certainly in health care, appraisal is a necessity, so the best way of addressing fear and anxiety is with knowledge, preparation, and practice. It may help the manager who is uneasy about appraisal to remember that appraisal is not the employee's favorite activity either. We might often have reason to wonder who dreads the upcoming performance appraisal more—the manager or the employee.

OBSTACLES TO PERFORMANCE APPRAISAL

There are other obstacles to performance appraisal in addition to the manager's and employee's possible dislike of the process.

In some organizations appraisal is not used to best effect, so managers view performance appraisal as little more than a paper-pushing, file-stuffing activity that is not especially relevant. Some appraisal instruments (that is, the required forms and instructions) have become so lengthy and complex that the sheer weight of the process becomes another source of dread for the department manager.

Given the way many systems are structured, especially those that relate pay increases to performance level, appraisal results must be converted to "scores" along the way. For some participants the performance appraisal becomes a "scorecard," and the process becomes competitive.

One ever-present problem is the difficulty of ensuring consistent application from manager to manager. Across-the-board consistency is important, especially in applying systems in which evaluation scores determine the amounts of pay increases. But differences are at times evident in that:

- Some managers are "hard" raters, rarely if ever giving outstanding scores or even scores above the middle of the scale
- Some managers are "soft" raters, consistently scoring all employees on the high side of the scale
- Some managers have a tendency to "cluster" their ratings, for instance grouping most employees in a narrow band around the middle of the scale
- Different managers often emphasize different parts of the system, with one, for example, leaning heaviest on quality of output and another placing greatest stress on interpersonal relationships.

Another obstacle of an extremely practical nature has arisen with the recent tendency toward "merger mania." Mergers and other forms of affiliation (as well as reengineering, downsizing, and organizational flattening) have left some managers with extremely large units with many employees. Some managers feel they do not have sufficient time to do justice to so many evaluations; this is often borne out when one discovers that the appraisals done first are the most thorough, while those done later are likely to have been rushed. Also, the manager responsible for a large number of employees may be hesitant to appraise because he or she may not be sufficiently familiar with all aspects of every employee's work.

Finally, older performance appraisal systems were often highly personality-based. Even though systems have changed, some long-time managers inappropriately tend to render personality judgments in appraising performance.

PERSONALITY-BASED EVALUATION: THE OLD WAY IS THE WRONG WAY

Earlier systems of performance appraisal tended to rely heavily on the assessment of personality characteristics. This resulted in evaluations that were largely if not entirely subjective. The old tendency in appraisal was much like the old tendency in pre-civil rights interviewing in that it encouraged more of a focus on what the employee *is* rather than what the employee *does* and how well it is done relative to some standard.

Following are some examples taken from a form used years ago for evaluating the performance of nonmanagerial employees. In each subsection the evaluator is given a choice of five statements and must check one that best describes the employee. After each, some commentary has been provided concerning the evaluation statements that were used. This exercise is undertaken specifically to demonstrate the weaknesses of personality-based appraisal.

I. ATTENDANCE
1. Punctuality
    ☐ Always on time
    ☐ Occasionally late
    ☐ Requires occasional reminding
    ☐ Often tardy; treats job as unimportant
    ☐ Always tardy

Commentary: In old evaluation systems, attendance was often the only item that was quantifiable. However, this instrument calls for subjectivity in assessing attendance. "Occasional" and "often" surely do not have the same meaning for all people, and "treats job as unimportant" is a completely unsubstantiated conclusion. Also, this uses two of the most dangerous words one can ever use in describing employee behavior: "always" and "never." Rarely if ever are they absolutely true.

2. Dependability
    ☐ Perfect since last rating
    ☐ Rarely absent
    ☐ Frequently absent, but for cause
    ☐ Poor record, requires counseling
    ☐ Unsatisfactory; work suffers

Commentary: Each of these statements is completely subjective except for the first one—if we can take "Perfect since last rating" to mean no absences in the intervening period. Again there are words that have no absolute meanings, such as "rarely," "frequently," etc. And the middle item suggests that the evaluator has to judge "dependability" according to whether an employee's absences are "for cause" or not, but this cannot be done factually without violating an employee's privacy; as long as the employee has called in according to policy, the manager must take each absence at face value.

II. PERSONAL QUALIFICATIONS
1. Appearance
   - ☐ Neat and in good taste
   - ☐ Neat but occasionally not in good taste
   - ☐ Sometimes careless about appearance
   - ☐ Untidy
   - ☐ Unsuitable for job

Commentary: All five items are highly subjective. What is "good taste," and who defines it? Again there are words of imprecise definition. And we can be sure that one person's "untidy" is another person's "casual." This entire subsection is out of line. If used in an evaluation, "appearance" should be brought up only in reference to an accepted dress code or set of professional standards of conduct.

2. Personality
   - ☐ Exceptionally pleasing, a decided asset
   - ☐ Makes good impression, wears well
   - ☐ Makes good first impression only; does not wear well
   - ☐ Makes fair impression only
   - ☐ Creates unfavorable impression

Commentary: We can say little more about this than to point out that each of the five statements contains imprecise terminology and that the entire "Personality" subsection is completely irrelevant to an employee performance appraisal.

III. ATTITUDE TOWARD JOB
1. Interest
   - ☐ Shows intense enthusiasm and interest in all work
   - ☐ Shows interest; enthusiasm is not sustained
   - ☐ Passive acceptance; rarely shows enthusiasm
   - ☐ Shows little or no interest
   - ☐ Dislikes work

Commentary: Although it is constantly attempted, no one can appropriately appraise (or, for that matter, discipline) an employee for "attitude." These five imprecise statements are useless in appraising an employee, and the final one, "dislikes work," is an unwarranted and insupportable conclusion (the first four, in using "shows," are at least anchored in observation).

2. Cooperation
   - ☐ Goes all out to cooperate with management and co-workers
   - ☐ Promotes cooperation and good will
   - ☐ Moderately successful in cooperating with others
   - ☐ Cooperates reluctantly and sometimes causes dissension
   - ☐ Uncooperative; often breeds trouble

Commentary: Many users of this system would likely have trouble differentiating between the first two statements. Once again, the more negative statements are arguable and could not be successfully defended if challenged.

IV. JOB PERFORMANCE
1. Accuracy
   - ☐ Rarely makes mistakes
   - ☐ Above average
   - ☐ Average
   - ☐ Below average
   - ☐ Highly inaccurate

Commentary: These are all essentially subjective unless the evaluator has available a quantified definition of "average" as it relates to the particular job. None of these statements is defensible without supporting data.

2. Neatness
   - ☐ Takes pride in appearance of work; has sense of neatness
   - ☐ Usually turns out neat work
   - ☐ Apparently lacks sense of neatness; needs reminding
   - ☐ Too often sacrifices neatness for quantity
   - ☐ Majority of work must be done over

Commentary: This subsection is one of the weakest in the system in that it all hinges on someone's subjective definition of "neat." And looking at the final statement, since "majority" literally means more than 50 percent, we might suggest that if someone whose work needs to be redone more than half the time has been allowed to remain long enough even to be evaluated, something is dreadfully wrong.

3. Quantity
   - ☐ Unusually high output; meets emergency demands well
   - ☐ Consistently turns out more than average
   - ☐ Finishes allotted amount
   - ☐ Does just enough to get by
   - ☐ Amount of work done is inadequate

Commentary: This is a particularly weak listing given that in many instances "quantity" is one of the most objectively measurable evaluation criteria available. There is of course imprecise language throughout, as well as the same sort of inconsistency found under "Neatness": If someone "does just enough to get by," it would suggest that one who did even less was not "getting by" and thus should not be there, making the final statement useless.

The foregoing is typical of the contents of systems of performance appraisal that relied almost exclusively on the evaluator's subjective judgments. Is it any wonder that a great many managers were uneasy with the appraisal process? A subjective assessment is merely an opinion when expressed by someone who is not qualified in the particular area of the judgment, and how many department managers are qualified to render personality judgments? Under these former approaches managers were required to make judgments they were not qualified to make and could not possibly defend, yet they knew these judgments could affect someone's employment.

Of course, such appraisals were probably as unsettling to the employee as they were to the manager. Few employees will willingly or readily agree with a manager's assessment if it includes negative subjective judgments that are in fact no more than the manager's opinions. Will an employee readily agree that he or she "creates (an) unfavorable impression," "often breeds trouble," or "cannot be depended upon"?

This kind of inappropriate performance appraisal was often formerly used in environments in which authoritarian management prevailed. In an authoritarian situation the evaluator could freely use personal opinions, unsupported judgments, and even personal biases on evaluations. The employees, if they wanted to keep on being employees, had no recourse other than to swallow their anger and get back to work.

WHAT, THEN, IS THE CORRECT APPROACH?

The appropriate way to truly appraise *performance* is to base the evaluation on what the employee *does*, not on what the employee *is* or *knows*. For decades it was traditional, for example, to have managers rate employees on a category called "job knowledge." In addition to being subjective, this sort of assessment revealed little or nothing of value. It is not job knowledge that matters; what really matters is how that knowledge is applied—that is, the results achieved.

The correct approach to appraisal—or at least the approach that is far more accepted today by evaluators and employees alike—is to base the evaluation on how well the employee is doing the job that he or she is expected to do. Preparation for this appraisal begins with consideration of the specific tasks that make up the job in question.

Solid Job Descriptions

A sound performance appraisal begins with a solid job description. The job description usually originates with the department manager, often with assistance from Human Resources (at least regarding form and format), and usually involves securing the input of the person who does the job.

Up-to-date job descriptions are necessary for a number of reasons, only one of which (but an important one) is their use in performance appraisal. To evaluate the employee on what he or she actually does, we require a clear picture of what is expected of that employee. We need to know the tasks to be performed and the results to be achieved so we have a baseline against which to compare observed performance.

In the language of health care performance appraisal in the 1980s and into the 1990s, we heard much about the need for evaluation to be "criteria-based." More recently the emphasis has turned to evaluation based on "competencies." We can rightly describe evaluation "criteria" as the requirements of the job description and describe "competencies" as "applied knowledge and skills" that fulfill the requirements of the job description. Whichever term is used, the net effect is the same as long as the employee is working according to an approved job description.

The primary shortcoming of many job descriptions is the extent of detail their writers attempt to capture. A lengthy, detailed job description leads to excessive length and detail in the performance appraisal. Most job descriptions need not be lengthy; for many entry-level jobs or nonprofessional positions, 9 or 10 lines describing the most time-consuming tasks in descending order (that is, with the most time-consuming duty listed first) is adequate. These few lines should be able to capture 90 to 95 percent of the job, which is sufficient for a job description for most uses. It does not pay to give a task that takes only a few minutes once each week the same space and attention as a task that takes two hours each day. Excessive detail places the manager at risk of paying as much attention to minor concerns as to major job requirements.

Exhibit 10-1 presents a sample job description for the position of nursing assistant. This job description was developed along the lines suggested, listing a few summary duties that admittedly do not encompass everything that might be done but that cover more than 90 percent of what the employee does on any given day. It would of course be relatively easy to break down the summarized duties into many more specific responsibilities (one sample nursing assistant job description reviewed during research for this chapter listed 68 distinctly separate tasks while another listed more than 90 duties grouped into several categories) yet still not capture all that might have to be done. If the evaluating manager knows the job and the employee as he or she should, the appropriate detail will emerge upon appraisal in those specific areas where attention is required. Multi-page, detailed job descriptions lead to multi-page, detailed performance appraisals that require more and more time to address. This simply adds more time and attention to creating and filing paper and detracts from time for people.

As noted in Chapter 7, How to Conduct a Legal—but Effective—Selection Interview, a job description should be one of the first considerations when a new job is being created, and an existing job description should be reviewed and updated when it becomes necessary to recruit for the position or when there are obvious changes in the job (such as new methods or equipment). Another good time to review job descriptions for current applicability is when preparing to do performance appraisals.

Once a current job description is in hand, attention should turn to how to measure performance against the task requirements or how to assess whether the employee's results are acceptable. It is usually possible to apply objective measures to some parts of most jobs. It is not always possible to measure everything that is done, but for most jobs

Exhibit 10-1 Sample Job Description

Department: Nursing

Position: Nursing Assistant, General Medical/Surgical

Grade: N-3   Job Code: 607

Reports to: Unit Manager (will on occasion report to designated nurse in charge).

Principal Duties (List in descending order of approximate percentage of time required):

1. Provides timely personal care of acceptable quality to patients in accordance with established policies, procedures, standards, and approved individualized care plans in manner mindful of patient privacy, comfort, and safety.
2. Performs routine treatments and other patient care as assigned, competently completing all assigned treatments during the scheduled shift. Also assists RN or LPN with nursing care and treatments as needed.
3. Assists RN or LPN in gathering data for patient assessment, including vital signs and height, weight, intake and output, and other measurements as applicable; demonstrates ability to recognize and report abnormal vital signs; demonstrates ability to properly collect and accurately label specimens.
4. Maintains positive interpersonal relationships with patients, visitors, and other staff while ensuring confidentiality of patient information and protection of patient privacy.
5. Maintains conscientious work habits consistent with the standards of the Nursing Department, specifically: documenting clearly and completely, managing assignments with normal supervision, completing duties within the assigned shift, accepting reassignment to other units as necessary, and responding favorably to reasonable requests to remain beyond the shift when needed.
6. Operates equipment and performs work in a safe manner, demonstrating proper body mechanics in lifting, pulling, pushing, carrying, etc.
7. Maintains the clinical and educational standards of the department: maintains CPR certification and demonstrates effective performance in "code" procedures; participates in unit and department in-service education activities; remains current with all continuing education requirements.
8. Observes the departmental standard for attendance and punctuality; calls in according to policy when absence or extended tardiness is unavoidable.
9. Maintains a professional appearance at all times in accordance with the hospital's dress code; exhibits a professional demeanor when dealing with patients, families, medical staff, and other employees.
10. Undertakes other assignments as directed by the unit manager or officially designated charge nurse.

it is possible to come up with something more concrete than a totally subjective assessment for many of the duties.

Sources of Standards and Measures

Measures of performance should address four key dimensions: productivity, quality, timeliness, and cost. Sources of performance standards include:

- *Detailed time-study and methods analysis.* Some of the most accurate standards can be developed using this approach. However, the process is time-consuming and costly, to the extent that this approach is suitable only for high-volume, highly repetitive activities (of which there are few in health care).
- *Predetermined motion-time systems.* Highly accurate standards can be developed using this approach, but it is also time-consuming and costly. This process is also most suitable for high-volume repetitive activities.
- *Work sampling.* Reasonably reliable standards can be established through work sampling. The process is time-consuming, but not nearly as costly as the above two means. Nevertheless, it requires special skills and a person who can be dedicated largely to developing standards. Work sampling is applicable to moderately repetitive activities and some occasional activities.
- *Benchmarks.* These are indicators of productivity that have either been developed through the experience of various organizations or published by interested organizations such as associations of health care organizations or technical or professional societies. Benchmarks are inexpensive, often available at no cost but sometimes acquired via purchased subscription to a statistical reporting service or through membership in an association. Benchmarks are readily applicable but usually not nearly as accurate as the "engineered standards" of the above three sources. Also, benchmarks can at times be misleading because the user often has no clear idea whether the method on which a benchmark is based is similar to the method used where the benchmark is to be applied.

Following are some examples of the kinds of indicators for which standards may be established or benchmarks acquired. As noted, these relate to productivity (or quantity), quality, time, and cost.

For Productivity (Quantity)
- Number of patients served per unit of time
- Number of items processed or produced per unit of time
- Number of cases handled per unit of time
- Percentage of employees participating
- Percentage of employees absent, tardy, etc.

For Quality
- Percentage of retakes (radiology) or test repeats (laboratory)
- Error rate
- Percentage of downtime (equipment out of service)
- Number of citations upon inspection or survey
- Percentage of work rejected
- Percentage of orders, bills, etc., without error

For Time
- Number or percentage of bills out within X days
- Number or percentage of deadlines missed
- Number of days to complete task or project
- Time elapsed, or turnaround time
- Number or percentage of requests answered within X days

For Cost
- Expense compared with previous period
- Percentage of variance from budget
- Cost per item, per order received, per bill processed, per patient contact, etc.
- Overtime cost compared with target
- Contract help cost compared with target

The benchmarks or other guides obtained from various sources are then associated with such indicators to become standards of measurement against which individual or even team or departmental performance can be assessed. A simple example that can apply to all employees is attendance. Say the organization's expectation is that three absences (call-ins, not scheduled time off) in a 12-month period is the normal or target for the employee population. Rather than hold to a rigid standard of three, a range is allowed such that the "standard" for attendance is "two to four absences." Therefore, the employee who had two, three, or four call-in absences during the year is considered to have met the standard. The employee who was absent five or more times fell short of the standard; the employee who was absent once or not at all exceeded the standard.

The Use of Objectives

Some employees may be evaluated in part on how well they do in meeting certain objectives that resulted largely from previous evaluations. Objectives are best established jointly by employee and manager, with the manager ensuring that each objective is pertinent and the employee agreeing that each objective is fair and reasonable. Some appraisal processes, especially those applying mostly to technical, professional, or managerial employees, rely heavily on such objectives. Some objectives arise from weaknesses revealed during an evaluation; for example, an employee who fell below standard in processing bills might agree to work toward improving billing output by 20 percent by the next evaluation. Some objectives have to do with personal development; for example, an employee who aspires to greater responsibility may make completion of a course in public speaking an objective.

The appraisal approach based on management by objectives (MBO), largely applicable to managers and professionals, will consist largely of objectives negotiated between employee and immediate superior. Whatever the context of the use of objectives, however, an appropriate objective always includes an expression of *what*, *how much*, and *when*. Referring to one of the above examples, the complete objective for the bill processor might be: Improve my billing output (*what*) by 20 percent (*how much*) by the next evaluation (*when*). Without all three components, a supposed objective is not a legitimate objective.

Scale Points

A number of appraisal systems, especially older ones, call for the evaluator to measure or judge each evaluation criterion on some scale consisting of a number of gradations indicated by check-off boxes or blanks. Some actual examples:

- Five gradations: Unacceptable, Below Competent, Competent, Very Well, and Exceptional
- Eight boxes in a line, left end labeled "Low," right end labeled "High," with no designation on the boxes in between

- Eight columns simply numbered (1) through (8), with (8) being the highest rating
- A choice of rating someone (1) through (6), with (6) being the highest rating.
- Another five-point scale: (1) Definitely Unsatisfactory, (2) Substandard, but Making Progress, (3) Doing an Average Job, (4) Definitely Above Average, (5) Outstanding.

Many different evaluation scales have been employed, and most of them exhibit the same weaknesses in that they call for the evaluator not only to render subjective judgments but to render them along an arbitrary scale. It is tough enough to try to assess something as ethereal as "attitude" without also having to place one's assessment along a scale from 1 to 6, 7, or 8.

Experience with more modern appraisal systems has shown that a low, odd number of gradations works best. Some systems use five points; some of the more effective job description–based systems use only three points. Three points are more than sufficient in assessing performance. For each task on the job description there should be a standard or an expectation of behavior. The employee can then fall into only one of three places relative to the standard or expectation: failed to meet the standard, met the standard, or exceeded the standard. This three-point scale is especially appropriate in that a number of the standards or expectations can be expressed as acceptable ranges rather than specific numbers (as "one to three absences" in the earlier example).

"Average" vs. "Standard"

In many appraisal systems, "average" is used to describe what is supposedly desired performance (for example, the scale that places "doing an average job" in the center of the scale). However, we also frequently refer to "standards" and "standard performance." Far too often these terms are used interchangeably. But "average" and "standard" are not the same.

If we equate "average" with "standard," this suggests that as many as half of the employees are "below standard" and thus should probably not be employed. It is the intent of every reasonable appraisal system and every related improvement process to bring all employees to a level of "standard" or higher. Therefore, "standard" becomes the floor beneath which a level of performance cannot be tolerated.

Thus "standard" is the minimum acceptable level of performance. If that is the minimum and all are above it, then the true "average" of the group is well above "standard." Average may at times be a convenience in grouping scores once evaluations have been quantified, but "average" should not be used as a term to describe the expectations of the performance appraisal process.

Appraisal Timing

An employee's initial performance appraisal is typically at the end of the employment probationary period. This occurs at three months in many organizations and at six months in others. The probationary evaluation is done to determine whether the employee has learned the job adequately, after which the individual goes into the regular evaluation cycle. Although in some organizations performance appraisal is performed every six months, in most places it is an annual event.

There are two popular approaches to the annual appraisal: Everyone is evaluated at the same time once per year; or all employees are evaluated on or near their employment anniversary dates. Each approach has its proponents and its critics, and each has certain advantages and disadvantages.

The practice of evaluating all employees at the same time has its apparent advantages:

- Some consider it a distinct advantage that once evaluations are finished they are out of the way for essentially an entire year.
- Since all the reviews are done within a brief period of time, the application of evaluation criteria remains fairly consistent.
- Having all the appraisals accomplished at the same time can mesh closely with a pay-for-performance compensation system, allowing the accurate distribution of a predetermined amount of money because all appraisal scores are known at the same time.

On the negative side of an all-at-once appraisal system:

- It is a potentially massive task, consuming the manager's time and causing other important matters to go unattended for a period of time.
- The quality of the appraisals can diminish as the evaluator goes through the group, especially in departments with many people.

The proponents of anniversary date appraisal ordinarily contend:

- The appraisal workload is spread more or less evenly throughout the year, so there is no massive appraisal effort to contend with in a certain time period.
- Spreading the workload throughout the year ensures consistent quality of appraisals.

On the negative side of anniversary date appraisal, some will contend:

- The process requires constant monitoring by higher management and Human Resources rather than oversight for just a few weeks.
- Since evaluations are spread through the year, the appraisal task is never "caught up."
- The evaluator's interpretation and application of appraisal criteria are subject to change over time.
- If the process feeds a pay-for-performance system, it is extremely difficult to distribute a budgeted amount for increases because not all scores are known at once.

The performance appraisal should occur faithfully for every employee at the appointed time. However, much more than this is required between the manager and the employee. If an annual appraisal interview is the only time during the year that the manager and the employee meet to discuss the employee's performance, their relationship will be tenuous at best. The manager must maintain an ongoing relationship with each employee and be available to discuss work performance whenever circumstances warrant. It is a serious mistake to "save up" issues specifically for performance appraisal time.

Description of the Appraisal Procedure

An organization's performance appraisal process will ordinarily be described in a personnel policy and procedure manual. This document will reflect the features of the organization's appraisal process and delineate various responsibilities for the various stages of the process. As part of the policy and procedure manual, this description should be available for reference by employees at any time.

Exhibit 10-2 presents a model policy and procedure for an appraisal process based on anniversary date appraisal.

Exhibit 10-2   Model Policy and Procedure: Performance Appraisal

It is the policy of the Hospital to provide a formal performance appraisal for each employee at least once each year. The purposes of the appraisal program are to:

- Maintain or improve performance in the job the employee presently holds
- Assist in employee development by providing learning and growth opportunity for those wishing to advance
- Assist the Hospital in identifying individuals with advancement potential.

Performance appraisal applies to various employees as follows:

1. Newly hired employees:
   - The initial appraisal will occur at the end of the initial three- (3) month probationary period.
   - The second appraisal will occur three (3) months following the probationary appraisal.
   - The following appraisal will occur six (6) months later, or on approximately the employee's first anniversary of employment.
2. Employees promoted or transferred:
   - The initial appraisal conducted in an employee's new position will occur at either three (3) months or six (6) months, depending on the learning period established for the particular position.
   - Following successful completion of the learning period, the employee will revert to the normal appraisal scheduled per 3, below.
3. All employees:
   - Once having successfully completed the first year of employment or the learning period following promotion or transfer, each employee will be subject to appraisal on approximately the anniversary of his or her employment.

General Provisions of the Performance Appraisal Program:

- Appraisals in addition to those indicated in the foregoing may be instituted by the department manager when either a significant deterioration or a marked improvement in performance is evident.
- Regular communication with employees concerning performance is essential. Continuing positive communication can assist in motivating and reinforcing outstanding performance, which is the objective of the appraisal process. Regular communication

continues

**Exhibit 10-2   Model Policy and Procedure: Performance
            Appraisal** (continued)

may also call attention to specific needs for improvement in performance, and immediately addressing areas of need will help prevent them from emerging as major problems at formal appraisal time.
*   An appropriate performance appraisal should:
    1. Provide the employee with guidance in growing and developing as a performer
    2. Provide the manager with a means for personalizing management guidance to the individual employee
    3. Provide the employee with direction consistent with that appropriate for pursuing the objectives of the department and the organization
    4. Provide the manager with a way of assessing an employee's performance and placing a value of the effectiveness of this performance
    5. Result in a more effective work force, as individuals tend to perform more appropriately when they know what is expected of them and they are able to gauge their performance against periodic measurement.

The following procedure applies to the performance appraisal process:

1. Approximately 30 days in advance of an employee's scheduled appraisal date, Human Resources will send the department manager an appraisal form for the employee with the heading information completed.
2. The employee's job description provides the pattern for the appraisal. Before attempting the appraisal the manager should ascertain that the job description is complete and accurate. If necessary, the job description should be updated at this time, before the appraisal is attempted.
3. In addressing the appraisal, for exempt (salaried) professional, technical, and supervisory employees the manager should assess performance primarily against the actual accomplishment of duties and responsibilities as enumerated in the job description. Nonexempt (hourly) employees should be assessed primarily on the timely and accurate completion of assigned duties.
4. As appropriate, and provided that plans and objectives were enumerated when the previous appraisal was discussed, consideration should also be given to employee growth and

continues

Exhibit 10-2 Model Policy and Procedure: Performance Appraisal (continued)

development and improvements in performance that might have occurred since the previous appraisal.

5. Objective, quantifiable measures of performance should be applied wherever possible. For example, the Hospital's standards for attendance and punctuality may be applied, as may the output standards available in some departments. For duties for which no objective measure of performance is available, the manager should be able to reasonably describe a "standard" expectation and indicate why, in his or her judgment, the employee did or did not meet or exceed the expectation.

6. Once completed, each appraisal must be submitted for review and approval by the next highest level of management.

7. When higher management approval of an appraisal has been secured, the manager may schedule the employee for an appraisal conference. Every effort should be made to accomplish this conference no more the five (5) working days before or after the employee's anniversary date.

8. The manager is urged to follow good interviewing practices in conducting the appraisal conference by providing adequate time, privacy, reasonable comfort, and freedom from interruptions.

9. As appropriate (primarily for technical, professional, and supervisory employees), the manager and employee will jointly determine goals, objectives, and development plans to be pursued during the period preceding the next appraisal. As necessary, they should achieve agreement on interim dates on which to examine progress between appraisals.

10. At the completion of the appraisal conference, the employee should be asked to sign the appraisal document to acknowledge having discussed it and received a copy. If necessary, the employee may be reminded that signing the appraisal is simply acknowledgment and does not necessarily mean agreement with all that it says. The employee may add comments of disagreement or agreement in the appropriate space on the appraisal form.

11. Should an employee refuse to sign his or her appraisal, the manager should so note the fact on the form. If in the manager's judgment the employee is in strong disagreement with the appraisal and may appeal or take other action, the manager may want to secure another party as witness to the refusal to sign and so indicate on the form.

continues

> **Exhibit 10-2 Model Policy and Procedure: Performance Appraisal** (continued)
>
> 12. Following the conference the completed appraisal is distributed as follows:
>   * Original to Human Resources
>   * Copy to employee
>   * Copy retained by manager.

THE APPRAISAL INTERVIEW

The overwhelming majority of performance appraisal systems call for each employee to receive a personal appraisal interview. We can go so far as to say that this appraisal interview is a *must;* the manager's appraisal responsibility is not completed until after each employee has had the opportunity to discuss his or her appraisal in detail. With regard to the appraisal interview, the manager should:

* Make certain the appraisal interview occurs when it is supposed to. Few occurrences in the workplace can raise apprehensions and uncertainties faster than appraisals that run later than scheduled.
* Schedule sufficient time for the meeting. The appraisal interview may seem routine to the manager, but it is one of the most important annual events for many employees, so it should never seem rushed.
* As with any kind of interview, arrange for privacy and freedom from interruptions.
* Give the employee some advance notice, at least a few days, so that he or she can be properly prepared.
* If the review in question is of the kind that involved objectives as well as ratings, review the objectives before the interview and prepare to discuss them.
* Again if it is the kind of review that involves objectives, come into the interview with some ideas to present to the employee or some suggestions to put forth concerning objectives for the coming cycle.
* If you have determined that some area of improvement or correction is needed, during the course of the interview help the employee work out what he or she should do to effect correction.

- In delivering praise as well as criticism, be certain to address specifics; never offer generalizations (this goes for both the written appraisal and the appraisal interview).
- Should follow-up on objectives or any other open issue be indicated, before concluding the interview reach agreement with the employee regarding when you will meet again.
- In concluding the interview, ask the employee to sign the appraisal form to acknowledge receipt (*not* necessarily to indicate agreement). Should the employee decline to sign, proceed as you would when an employee refuses to sign a disciplinary notice and note the refusal on the form.
- Supply the employee with a copy of the evaluation.

As in any other kind of interview, from the manager's perspective the most important parts of an appraisal interview occur while the evaluator is listening, not speaking.

In some instances, because of overlapping shift assignments and split-shift responsibilities of managers, an employee may be reporting to different supervisors at various times. The primary input to such an employee's appraisal must come from the manager who directly supervises the employee most of the time, supplemented with input from other involved supervisors. The manager who provides the majority of direct supervision should also be the one who conducts the appraisal interview.

Neither the written performance appraisal nor the appraisal interview should hold surprises for the employee; there should never be a feeling of "Gotcha!" caused by something critical coming out of the blue. The employee should know fairly well where he or she stands with the manager at all times; it is the manager's responsibility to ensure that this is the case.

SELF-APPRAISAL

Depending on how and by whom it is used, self-appraisal can be a productive part of a performance appraisal system. However, self-appraisal is not for everyone; some employees are intimidated by it, and some are apprehensive, fearing what they see as the possible consequences of rating themselves "too high" or "too low." Self-appraisal is probably most appropriate for higher-level technical employees, professionals, supervisors, and managers. This is not to say that self-appraisal cannot have its advantages when used with many rank-and-file employees, but it is within the ranks that we find the most uneasiness about the process and suspicions of its intent.

Under self-appraisal some people tend to rate themselves either higher or lower than may be appropriate. Research has repeatedly shown that the majority of employees rate themselves no higher, and frequently lower, than their supervisors rate them.

Self-appraisal best fits into the overall performance appraisal process as follows:

- The employee does the self-appraisal, and the manager writes up the employee's performance appraisal. These tasks occur completely *separately.* The employee should not be given the manager's appraisal before completing the self-appraisal, and the manager should not see the self-appraisal before completing his or her appraisal of the employee. There should be no possibility of one appraisal biasing the other.
- The form used for the self-appraisal can be the same form used by the manager for the primary appraisal, or it may be a simpler version of that form. The self-appraisal need not be as detailed as the primary appraisal, but it should address the same major job description criteria.
- The employee brings the self-appraisal to the appraisal interview with the manager. This should be the first time that both parties see both appraisals.
- At the beginning of the appraisal interview the two appraisals are compared item by item, with the participants making note of any areas in which the two assessments diverge appreciably.
- The divergence of evaluations highlights the most important aspect of the self appraisal's use: It serves to focus the discussion where it is likely to be needed most. For example, say a manager and an employee go through an evaluation consisting of eight job description requirements. Upon meeting, they discover that their ratings on six of the eight criteria are fairly close, but on the remaining two criteria they are far enough apart to raise some concerns that need exploring. Thus, the self-appraisal has been able to focus the discussion on what are potentially the most important points relating to the perceptions of this employee's performance.

Surely self-appraisal is not appropriate for every appraisal situation and is not necessarily helpful in some instances. However, in appraising those employees who are required to exercise some amount of independent discretion and judgment—as do the technical, professional, and managerial employees who make up a large part of the health care work force—self-appraisal can be a constructive adjunct to the performance appraisal system. Also, self-appraisal draws employees more deeply into the appraisal process and makes it much more of a participative activity.

TEAM APPRAISALS

During the recent couple of decades we have heard a great deal about the use of teams of various kinds and seen increasing interest in team building and in developing ways of enhancing team productivity. In spite of this ever-increasing focus on teams, however, for the most part performance appraisal processes remain individually focused.

Individual evaluations rendered in a team environment can be troublesome because they tend to:

- Undermine teamwork by stressing individual competitiveness
- Encourage competitive individuals to circumvent team requirements for individual gain
- Fail to encourage an open, problem-solving environment.

Individual performance appraisals do not support team-building in that they lack a means of dealing with the effects of the individual on the group or the group on the individual. Individual appraisals can be a drag on effective team building.

Teams can of course be appraised as teams, but there is a glaring weakness inherent in doing so. That weakness lies in the inevitable differences that exist among individuals—some people will always perform better or worse than others. A properly managed team should be able to use the various strengths of all its members, but it is clear that a team is no place for either single "stars" or individual slackers.

As with individual performance appraisals, team evaluation requires criteria and standards—but these must be constructed specifically in terms of team performance. In some organizations, group or team appraisals are used as a supplement to, rather than a replacement for, individual performance appraisals. This could be the most workable solution to the team-versus-individual dilemma; even in well-functioning teams there will always be some individuals who are more or less productive than others.

Thus, although the emphasis on teams and team performance continues to increase, the overwhelming majority of our reward and recognition systems are focused on the individual. This reinforces the need to appraise both team performance and individual performance.

THE APPRAISAL FORM

The major shortcoming of many performance appraisal systems, as well as the job description processes they are linked to, is that they attempt to capture far too much detail. The appraisal systems that usually generate the greatest amount of frustration and resistance with managers use forms that are many pages long and require dozens, sometimes hundreds, of separately detailed assessments. One sample reviewed for this chapter, the appraisal of a nursing assistant, consisted of nine pages containing 94 detailed assessments divided into seven categories—all of which covered just the organizational requirements of a nursing assistant; several pages of unit-specific criteria had to be addressed as well in each nursing unit. It is doubtful that any conscientious manager would look forward to doing a number of these, especially when we consider that in the organization this sample was taken from, the registered nurse appraisal was even longer and more detailed.

A lengthy, detailed appraisal form creates extraneous work for appraisers and rapidly fills personnel files with paper. Some organizations have tried to compensate for this by filing only a summary document which, upon reference, had to be interpreted using an external key. Once filed, however, an appraisal should be a self-contained record that can be understood on its own should it ever have to be referenced.

Any performance appraisal form than runs longer than two or three pages should be considered suspect; moreover, the few pages that are used should have as few detailed spaces as possible. A peculiar two-sided problem occasionally arises with fill-in-the-spaces types of appraisal forms:

- Not all the blocks or spaces will apply to every person's evaluation, but some appraisers feel they should write *something* in every available space.
- Some of the spaces are not large enough to contain all that should be said about some particular items, but some appraisers will simply fill the available space and stop.

No particular appraisal form is precisely the right form for all uses. Some organizations have gone so far as to have two or three or more different forms to be used for evaluating different kinds of staff. For example, one health care organization, a hospital in the 400- to-500-bed range, maintained and used four separate appraisal forms—one each for hourly employees, managers, registered nurses, and professional staff other than nurses. If there seems to be an advantage to using different forms or even different systems for different classes of employees, so be it. But all should employ a common face sheet or heading information section that displays final evaluation results and scores in a manner consistent with all others.

Although no single appraisal form is best for all uses, the most useful forms are those that have a minimum of fill-in spaces and a maximum of open writing space.

Whether by using a triplicate form or simply by using a photocopier, each performance appraisal should be generated in three copies. The manager is generally responsible for seeing that these copies get to the appropriate people following the appraisal interview and obtaining the employee's signature: original to Human Resources for the official personnel file, a copy for the manager's files, and a copy for the employee.

Exhibits 10-3 and 10-4 are examples of performance appraisal forms similar to some in actual use. Exhibit 10-3 is generic, an open format that can conceivably be used along with any number of different job descriptions. The rating scale is the simplest in common use—three levels, to indicate whether the employee has not met the standard, met the standard, or exceeded the standard. The numbers attached to these three levels of performance are simply a convenience for converting the appraisal results into an overall "score" for whatever use it may be put (for example, determining the amount of a merit increase). Exhibit 10-4 is considerably more specific to the point of being written for a particular position. As in the previous example, this approach uses a three-point scale with the "standard" or expectation lying at the "2" in the middle. This exhibit also allows for the potential use of "weighting"; if duty number 1, for example, is considered twice as important or twice as time-consuming as any of the others, it might be given a weight of "2," meaning that it will count twice as heavily as the others in the final average score. Note also that the approach taken in Exhibit 10-4 suggests that it is often possible, even advisable, to combine a job description and a performance appraisal in a single document.

Exhibit 10-3   Generic Performance Appraisal

Employee Name: _____ ID No. _____

Department: _____ Hire Date _____

Job Title/Grade _____ Job Date _____

	Job Description Requirement	**Rating**		
No.	**Task and Expectation (Standard)**	**Not Met**	**Met**	**Exceeded**
___	_____	___	___	___
___	_____	___	___	___
___	_____	___	___	___
___	_____	___	___	___
___	_____	___	___	___
___	_____	___	___	___
___	_____	___	___	___
___	_____	___	___	___
___	_____	___	___	___
___	_____	___	___	___
___	_____	___	___	___
___	_____	___	___	___
___	_____	___	___	___
___	_____	___	___	___
___	_____	___	___	___
___	_____	___	___	___
___	_____	___	___	___
___	_____	___	___	___
___	_____	___	___	___
___	_____	___	___	___

continues

Exhibit 10-3   Generic Performance Appraisal (continued)

Scoring: For each "Not Met," score "0." For each "Met," score "2."

For each "Exceeded," score "4."

Totals --   _____   _____   _____

Average* ---   _____

*   — Average 2.0 equals standard performance.

Greater than 2.0 equals exceptional performance.

Less than 2.0 means improvement is required.

Manager's Comments:

Employee's Comments:

Date of Discussion: _____

Employee Signature: _____

Manager Signature: _____

LEGAL IMPLICATIONS OF PERFORMANCE APPRAISAL

In health care, performance appraisal has become a regulatory necessity. The Joint Commission on Accreditation of Healthcare Organizations (JCAHO) looks for appraisal in the personnel files during its periodic surveys, as do many of the state health departments. Performance appraisal should of course be pursued as a means of employee development, but it also must be done to avoid being cited for deficiencies.

Although there are legal risks associated with doing and retaining performance appraisals, on balance it appears that the legal risks of *not* doing so are greater.

When an employee is terminated for reasons related to job performance, or is perhaps selected for layoff in preference to another employee, if the action is contested (especially through an external advocacy agency or court), performance appraisal documents in the per-

Exhibit 10-4 Performance Appraisal for a Specific Position

Employee Name: _____ ID No. _____
Department: ___Communications (Mail Room)_ Hire Date _____
Job Title/Grade _Driver-Mail Clerk/m-4_____ Job Date _____

Summary: Performs messenger duties that require driving hospital vehicles to various locations to pick up and deliver mail. Is also required to maintain and assist in the operation of mailroom equipment.

Requirements: Six (6) months clerical experience or direct experience in mailroom operations, ability to communicate in English sufficiently to perform the duties of the job, and a valid driver's license with a driving record free of moving violations.

	Weight	Score
1. Drives vehicles to deliver mail and packages to various locations.		
a. Delivers morning and afternoon mail within 1-1/4 hours of signing the courier log sheet, measured by quarterly review of log	_____	1 2 3
b. Performs special courier trips as requested, measured by observation.		1 2 3
c. Informs supervisor of vehicle or traffic problems upon return, measured by observation.		1 2 3
Comments:		

	Weight	Score
2. Picks up and delivers from/to post office.	_____	
a. Maintains morning mail schedule by picking up first-class and bulk mail from post office between 8:00 AM and 8:00 PM.		1 2 3
b. Maintains afternoon schedule by delivering stamped mail and picking up additional mail between 1:00 and 1:30 PM at post office, as observed.		1 2 3
c. Delivers afternoon mail to post office between 4:30 and 5:00 PM, as measured by observation.		1 2 3
Comments:		

continues

Exhibit 10-4 Performance Appraisal for a Specific Position (continued)

	Weight	Score
3. Operates mailing machine to apply postage.	_____	
a. Applies correct postage per current rates, as observed by supervisor.		1 2 3
b. Signs and completes internal postage voucher per department policy, as observed by supervisor.		1 2 3
c. Places all stamped mail in trays or bags for delivery to post office, as observed by supervisor.		1 2 3

Comments:

	Weight	Score
4. Reports vehicle mileage to supervisor and ensures vehicle upkeep.	_____	
a. Completes mileage log before and after each vehicle use, as measured by quarterly review of log.		1 2 3
b. Maintains clean vehicle by using car wash ticket each Friday immediately following morning delivery, as observed by supervisor.		1 2 3
c. Follows all policies governing vehicle use, as observed by supervisor.		1 2 3

Comments:

	Weight	Score
5. Assists with office machines and performs other duties.	_____	
a. Clears jams and resolves other minor copier problems following posted guidelines, as observed by supervisor.		1 2 3
b. Ensures that supplies for copiers and fax machines are maintained at reasonable levels, as observed by supervisor.		1 2 3
c. Locks mail room offices at 4:30 PM each day. Opens offices at 8:00 AM each day (standard = no more than 2 to 4 exceptions per year), as observed by supervisor		1 2 3

Comments:

sonnel file will become a central concern. For example, assume Employee A is laid off and Employee B, who does the same work and is similarly situated to A, is retained. The reason given for the choice is that "B is the better performer." If A contests the action, the contention that B is the better performer had better be borne out by appraisals in the two employees' personnel files. If this cannot be established by documentation, it may then be assumed that Employee A is a victim of discrimination or other personal bias.

Performance appraisals frequently figure prominently in wrongful discharge litigation. Whenever there is even a chance that any discharge was based wholly or in part on substandard performance, a wrongful discharge claim may be filed and information will be sought in the appraisal records in the personnel file. Thus, many wrongful discharge lawsuits are an outgrowth of inadequate performance appraisal procedures.

The largest number of legal complaints centered on performance appraisal issues involve alleged violations of individual rights as specified under Title VII of the Civil Rights Act of 1964. The second largest number of such complaints deal with alleged violations of the Age Discrimination in Employment Act (ADEA). Performance appraisal records may be examined closely if performance is used as a criterion in determining who will go in a large layoff or planned reduction in force (RIF), especially if there appears to be a disparate impact on any group or class of employee—which is a common complaint arising from the layoff of older workers.

Although there is no way to avoid some subjective assessment in the majority of performance appraisals, these are best kept to a minimum. By all means, always avoid potentially defamatory comments; keep insults, name-calling, and unsupported negative commentary out of every appraisal. Whenever entering negative assessments, cite provable specifics whenever possible.

The organization is not legally obligated to have a performance appraisal system. Once a system is put in place, however, the employer may be seen as having created an implied contract with employees to use the system as established and described.

The performance appraisal system should be sufficiently formal to have published instructions for accomplishing appraisals. These instructions, plus any evidence that can be presented concerning the training of appraisers in the system's use, can be helpful in defending the appraisal system against charges of discrimination.

THE ROLE OF HUMAN RESOURCES

The Human Resources department is usually the custodian of the performance appraisal system. HR's role in performance appraisal will ordinarily involve:

- Monitoring the state of job descriptions and evaluation criteria to ensure that these are always up-to-date and currently applicable.
- Designing the appraisal system. Ideally, system design or modification should be a joint effort of HR and a number of managers of both line and support activities.
- Scheduling the various steps in the process, such as establishing dates for forms to go out, appraisals to be written and discussed with employees, and completed appraisals to be submitted to HR.
- Providing forms, lists, and time schedules to the department managers as needed. In a system under which employees are evaluated on anniversary dates, someone in HR will constantly monitor the system and send out forms and reminders as employees' anniversary dates occur.
- Monitoring the incoming appraisals for completeness and consistency. Under some appraisal systems, appraisers are required to have their evaluations reviewed by the next level of management before they are discussed and submitted.
- Holding classes for evaluators, providing both original appraisal training and perhaps refresher training every year (if the organization does not have a separate education function). HR will also respond to evaluator's questions about system application.
- Following up to get evaluations completed within the proper time.
- Filing completed evaluations in individual personnel files, and addressing employees' questions and grievances about the appraisal process.

The next-to-last item above, following up on appraisal completion, represents an often stressful issue between line managers and Human Resources. The manager may not place high priority on what may be seen as a not particularly essential process, as well as feel pressures of too much to do and too little time to do it; HR, on the other hand, must follow higher management's mandate to keep the system moving. Timely appraisals are always important, and they become crucial under some of the all-at-once approaches that depend on having all scores in place for determining the distribution of merit pay increases. Nevertheless, HR's follow-up role sometimes causes department managers to view performance appraisal as "HR's system" or "just more of HR's paperwork."

AN ESSENTIAL PROCESS

The greatest part of most employees' performance is satisfactory or better; rarely are an individual's results completely or even largely unacceptable. Yet some managers neglect to express appreciation of an employee's successes but instead focus on failures and weaknesses, seeming to take the good for granted. This tendency to focus on the unsatisfactory simply reinforces the reputation of performance appraisal as a negative process.

Human Resources alone cannot guarantee a successful appraisal process, nor can even HR and a number of conscientious department managers working together do so. A critical element in the success of performance appraisal is the extent to which top management supports the process. Far too often top management simply says "Do it" to those down the hierarchy and fails to participate in any substantive manner. Lack of visible top management support increases the risk of appraisal becoming a meaningless routine. Many organizations, surely all health care organizations of any size, have performance appraisal systems. However, just because there *is* a system is no guarantee that performance appraisal in the organization is carried out effectively.

Discussion Points

1. Explain the essential difference between "average" and "standard" as these terms are used in performance appraisal, and describe how one of them is frequently used erroneously.
2. Over the years a number of authors of management material have recommended the complete abolition of performance appraisal. Provide three specific reasons why performance appraisal must continue as a process in the modern health care organization.

3. Consider an employee who always performs satisfactorily but has little or no opportunity to improve, and can go no higher in the organization and does not aspire to do so. Explain why it is considered necessary to continue periodically appraising this employee's performance.

4. Discuss why the appraisal of employee performance is frequently described as one of many department managers' least favorite responsibilities.

5. Discuss why it is so strongly recommended that all appraisal processes avoid addressing employees' personality characteristics? Shouldn't we want employees to convey "proper attitudes"?

6. Explain why it is appropriate practice to begin addressing an employee's performance with a review and update of the job description.

7. Provide two or three examples of some kind of work activity for which you could conceivably provide workable "standards."

8. Identify the three essential elements of an objective and explain why any stated objective is unworkable without all three present.

9. Explain why it is now frequently recommended that as few scale points as practical (often three and rarely more than five) be used in a rating-scale appraisal system.

10. Explain why it is extremely important to ensure that employee appraisals occur when they are scheduled to occur.

11. Describe a particular work group—it can be real or hypothetical—and make a case that either supports or opposes involving this group in mandatory self-appraisal.

12. Describe the primary shortcoming of team appraisal and suggest an approach to avoiding this shortcoming and still appraising on a team basis.

13. Explain why the Human Resources Department is a reasonable place from which to coordinate the organization's performance appraisal process.

14. One of the appraisal-related problems surfacing most often is the frequent lack of consistency in scoring from one manager to another. Explain how you would attempt to address this problem.

15. Describe the manner in which past appraisals of performance can influence the outcomes of certain employment-related legal actions.

CHAPTER 11

Addressing Problems before Taking Corrective Action

This chapter—

- Emphasizes the value and importance of preventing employee problems whenever possible
- Suggests that a key to preventing chronic absenteeism and tardiness is the manager's visible attention to both
- Addresses matters of employee privacy and confidentiality that often lead to conflict between individuals and organizations
- Reviews the legal steps that have been taken to protect employees' individual privacy
- Advises the department manager on how to respond to legal orders such as subpoenas, summonses, and warrants
- Reviews the organization's legal posture with respect to searches of employees' desks and lockers
- Reviews issues of access to employee personnel records, including the special status of employee health records
- Surveys different organizations' positions regarding personal relationships in the workplace
- Addresses the causes and possible prevention of violence in the workplace
- Recognizes the power of employee participation and involvement in avoiding potential problems
- Addresses counseling as an essential management skill for preventing certain circumstances from becoming genuine problems and for solving smaller problems before they become larger.

PREVENTION WHEN POSSIBLE

It goes without saying that the best time to address a problem is before it becomes a problem. We cannot readily anticipate difficulty occurring in specific forms at particular times, but by developing an awareness of a few areas of sensitivity and learning how to spot certain signs of trouble, the manager can catch many problems and would-be problems at their early stages.

It is not necessary to repeat what was said about discipline in Chapter 9, The Health Care Manager and Employee Problems, but an example from that chapter concerning absenteeism clearly illustrates the value of proactive prevention. The organization's policy concerning absences says that five instances of unexcused absence in a 12-month period or less call for the start of disciplinary action. Say you become aware that a particular employee has just been absent for the fourth time in eight months. Do you keep an eye on the employee and as soon as absence number five occurs, jump on the person with the start of disciplinary action? Why let it go that far if there might be something that you can do about it—something that might be easier for you and easier on the employee than taking disciplinary action? Take the employee aside and attempt to do something about his or her absenteeism before formal action becomes necessary. Exercise prevention whenever possible.

Concerning employee tardiness as well as absenteeism, an important aspect of problem prevention is the department manager's visible attention to both. If they can see the manager's attention to these problem areas, some employees will be deterred from abusing these particular work rules.

This chapter touches on a few of the more significant areas that can present problems for the manager in which conscientious and common-sense management can help minimize or avoid problems. The chapter concludes with a discussion of employee counseling, probably the most common approach to addressing potential problems before they become serious.

EMPLOYEE PRIVACY AND CONFIDENTIALITY

Issues of employee privacy and confidentiality loom large in today's work organizations, including health care organizations. Human Resources professionals are quite familiar with what has come to be a nearly constant tug-of-war between employee privacy and the right to know—that is, individual rights versus business need.

The rights of the individual to privacy and confidentiality have been a growing concern in our society for some time. In 1949 the novelist George Orwell delivered a stark warning of what could lie in the future in his landmark science fiction work, *1984*. Fortunately, many events have not occurred as Orwell fictionalized, but it was his work that gave us the now all-encompassing term used to describe government and its seemingly ever-expanding oversight of our lives: Big Brother. We fear that in a number of respects, Big Brother is watching over us.

Privacy and the Changing Times

There is an increasingly strong belief in society concerning an individual's right to privacy, and increasing apprehension about how the government might use the information it gathers about individuals. This concern stems from a number of reasons:

- Government seems to be regularly intruding deeper into peoples' lives with more and more laws and increasing demands for information.
- Businesses are perceived as seeking to know more about the people they employ.
- Since the horrifying events of September 11, 2001, the government has been responding to a perceived need to more closely screen individuals allowed into the country.
- Advancing and expanding computer technology is making the collection, storage, and retrieval of personal information easier.

Increasingly aware of their rights, employees are coming to expect that their privacy will be protected. At the same time, organizations are requesting an increasing amount of information about their employees for use in making decisions about hiring, promotions, benefits, and security. When people seek employment, organizations want information about past and present employers and other references. Depending on what the potential job entails, the application process may involve detailed security screening. Employees continue to grow increasingly sensitive to the issue of privacy rights, but at the same time they perceive that the organization is digging continually deeper into their personal lives. Many individuals believe that most organizations that collect information about them ask for more personal information than they legitimately need.

The right to privacy can be broadly stated as follows: "It is the right to be free from the unwarranted appropriation of one's personality, the publicizing of one's private affairs with which the public has no legitimate concern, or the wrongful intrusion into one's private activities, in such a manner as to outrage or cause suffering, shame or humiliation to a person of ordinary sensibilities."[1]

Consider individual privacy versus drug testing. Rights are continually giving way to perceived needs for drug testing, especially for people in occupations having responsibility for public health and safety. Consider also AIDS and HIV testing. This represents a constant collision of individual rights with the need to know of patients and coworkers. This particular controversy was largely responsible for health care adopting universal precautions under which all bodily fluids are regarded as potentially hazardous.

Many organizations once routinely used polygraph testing to screen potential employees and to make random checks of employees. Reaction to such growing intrusions eventually led to passage of the Employee Polygraph Protection Act of 1988.

Overall, an increasing number of issues in which employee information is a concern to management come down to the matter of business needs versus employees' expectations of privacy.

Legislation Affecting Privacy

Over the past few decades, employees have developed a stronger voice in how they fare in the workplace, and the government has responded. Large amounts of personal information were formerly requested on job applications and in employment interviews, but anti-discrimination laws now restrict the information that employers can request (see Chapter 7, How to Conduct a Legal—but Effective—Selection Interview, and Chapter 3, The Legal Framework of Present-Day Human Resources).

Title VII of the Civil Rights Act of 1964 was the first major law to have a significant bearing on individual privacy. The next major attack on this issue resulted in passage of the Privacy Act of 1974. Officially covering only agencies of the federal government but often regarded as a standard for other employers, this legislation:

- States that an agency may obtain and retain only information that is relevant and necessary to accomplish its official purposes
- Requires that as much essential information as possible come directly from the individual (rather than from secondary sources)
- Ensures record confidentiality
- Guarantees an employee's right to examine his or her personnel file
- Requires that no information be disclosed without the employee's consent.

In addition to providing a reasonable model for employers, the Privacy Act has served as a model for many states' privacy laws. Most states now have privacy laws that:

- Allow employees to know that a personnel file is maintained, and to examine it at will
- Permit employees to enter information in their files to clarify whatever they may consider to be inaccurate.

The Polygraph Protection Act of 1988 proclaimed the practice of routinely administered lie detector tests to be an invasion of privacy. This Act:

- Prohibits the use of lie detectors in most screening situations
- States that employees cannot be randomly tested during their term of employment
- Permits polygraph use if there is "reasonable suspicion" of involvement in workplace incidents resulting in economic loss or injury to the business
- Exempts government employers from coverage.

The Polygraph Protection Act does allow testing of certain employees in positions of responsibility for significant dollar value, including:

- Armored car employees
- Employees of alarm and security-guard firms

- Current and prospective employees of firms dealing with controlled substances.

The Fair Credit Reporting Act had the effect of limiting the extent to which an organization could delve into an individual's personal finances. This legislation:

- Regulates the conduct of consumer reporting agencies and users of consumer credit reports
- Prevents unjust damage from inaccurate or arbitrary information in credit reports
- Keeps employers from receiving reports about employees for other than certain specific work-related purposes.

Legal Orders

It is a relatively common practice for various agencies to serve subpoenas, summonses, and warrants to employees in the workplace. Many such orders are of course served at employees' homes, but frequently the officers attempt to accomplish service at the job site because no one can be found at an employee's last known address or no one is home during the work day. Some officers who serve such orders attempt to go directly to the employee's workplace. If they enter via Administration, they will probably be referred to Human Resources. In either Administration or HR, they will frequently ask directions to the employee's department. Although the practice may vary from one organization to another, a great many organizations prefer to have Human Resources arrange for such orders to be served in private and avoid unnecessary embarrassment to the individual.

The manager who becomes aware of an attempt to serve a legal order of any kind on an employee in the department should send the serving officer to Human Resources (as should any external request for information about an employee be referred to HR). Human Resources will arrange for the order to be served in private, or may perhaps even be able to accept it on behalf of the individual; this latter possibility depends on the kind of order it happens to be—HR is often able to accept on the person's behalf if the employee is being summoned as a witness in a legal proceeding.

Occasionally Human Resources will directly receive legal orders calling for certain employee information required in legal proceed-ings. Except for responding to legal orders, Human Resources will release no information to outside interests without securing a signed release from the affected employee.

Employee Searches

It will sometimes be considered necessary to conduct searches of areas within the facility, such as desks and lockers, that legitimately contain employees' personal property. The organization will ordinarily have a published policy governing such searches. Concerning employee searches:

- The organization should publicize the applicable policy so that employees know, for example, that there will be both for-cause and random searches.
- Steps should have been taken to ensure that the search policy can be justified (i.e., that there are good reasons for occasional searches).
- The search policy should be applied evenly and consistently, so there can be no perception of discrimination.
- Employee consent should be requested before a search. It is not legally required, but doing so can negate certain charges that might arise after the fact.
- Every search should be conducted discretely and with respect for individual person and property.

Access to Information

Issues of employee confidentiality always include questions of access to information. Once information is collected, who is entitled to see it? Although any number of arguments can be raised about the need to know, it is usually possible to judge what is a legitimate need by asking the question: What might be the result if this information is *not* made available?

As mentioned, employees now have the legally protected right to examine their personnel files and enter clarifications they believe necessary. The organization will ordinarily have a policy governing employee access to records, including the requirement that a file not leave the Human Resources department. Often the organization also stipulates that the file be reviewed in the presence of someone who can ensure that no material is removed.

An employee's personnel file may also be made available to certain managers who are considering the employee for a transfer opportunity. The need to know in this instance is a legitimate need to review the employment history of someone the manager may be considering for a position.

Every organization would be well advised to have a written policy governing the release of information concerning both employees and patients. If the department manager maintains files concerning employees in the department, this practice should be generally known; there should be no "secret" files on individuals.

Employee Health Records

Many organizations formerly kept employee health records related to worker's compensation, disability, and the like in employees' personnel files. However, most organizations have since concluded that documents relating to an employee's health or physical condition are medical records, and that medical records are subject to stricter rules of accessibility. That is, someone who might legitimately review a personnel record, such as a department manager considering a transfer candidate, need not have access to employee health records. Since this separate standard is applied to medical records, employee health records are now usually filed separately and are often retained by the employee health office in the manner in which a physician's office keeps patient records.

PERSONAL RELATIONSHIPS

Some organizations have rules governing personal relationships, particularly those of a romantic nature. It is not uncommon for an organization to prohibit employees being involved with each other or with employees of direct competitors. Generally, however, the employer can do nothing regarding an employee's off-duty conduct as long as it has no adverse effect on job performance or, in infrequent instances, on the organization's reputation.

Legitimate concerns may arise about the appearance of favoritism, and thus an increased likelihood of sexual harassment claims and employee unrest, when there are romantic relationships between management and nonmanagement employees. Related to such relationships, there may also be conflict between the employees' right to privacy and the organization's legal responsibility to prevent sexual harassment. The organization is particularly vulnerable when a member of management is involved; often the organization is held liable for sexual harassment by a manager even if the hierarchy above the manager knew nothing about what was occurring. As many organizations have discovered, a relationship that begins as consensual can go sour, leading to charges of sexual harassment.

Many organizations have a policy that prohibits placing one spouse under the supervision of the other, or even placing both spouses in the same department or group. Experience has shown that when these prohibitions are ignored, harmful perceptions can arise in the group. Little or nothing inappropriate may be occurring, but the possibility of discriminatory behavior can create such perceptions.

A rule against having spouses in a superior/subordinate relationship will ordinarily hold up under scrutiny, but prohibiting spouses in the same department may at times be challenged. Generally a no-spouse rule will prevail if it can be shown the rule is designed to avoid aggregation of family members, is applied evenly and consistently, and results in no adverse impact on either gender. However, uneven enforcement of this and similar rules can conceivably result in discrimination charges. Overall, all rules concerned with personal relationships are especially vulnerable to challenge under privacy and anti-discrimination laws.

SEXUAL HARASSMENT

The risk of sexual harassment charges extends far beyond the boundaries of failed consensual personal relationships.

Under the Civil Rights Act of 1964 and subsequently the Civil Rights Act of 1991, sexual harassment is a form of sex discrimination. Sexual harassment has become one of the two most frequently charged forms of discrimination for many employers (the other being age discrimination).

The generally increasing number of cases and the increasingly large monetary settlements involved make sexual harassment a concern of essentially every employer. The key position of every department manager relative to where and how sexual harassment most often occurs makes knowledge and awareness a must for the manager.

Sexual harassment consists of unwelcome sexual advances, demands, or requests for sexual favors, or other conduct of a sexual nature if:

- Acceptance of or submission to such conduct is either explicitly or implicitly a term or condition of employment
- Acceptance or rejection of such conduct is used as a basis for making employment-related decisions
- The conduct can be viewed as unreasonably interfering with work performance or creating an offensive or intimidating work environment (often referred to as a "hostile environment").

Sexual harassment can be as direct and blatant as offensive touching or direct sexual propositions, or it can be as indirect as sexually suggestive posters and calendars or sexually related humor (even a "dirty joke" overheard by someone who finds it offensive can constitute sexual harassment). A list of specific examples of behavior that could be interpreted as sexual harassment could fill several pages without covering all the possibilities. Moreover, some particular types of behavior might constitute sexual harassment at one time but not at another time. For example, it is ordinarily not considered sexual harassment for an individual to ask a co-worker for a date. But if the person who is asked declines and yet the asker repeatedly asks for a date, this can be construed as sexual harassment. Often the determination of whether some type of conduct is or is not considered sexual harassment is in the mind of the perceiver. Behavior that is judged to be sexual harassment is generally unwelcome, unwanted, and repeated.

Most organizations have a policy that prohibits sexual harassment and also specifically prohibits retaliation against anyone complaining of such harassment. It is the department manager's responsibility to know the sexual harassment and anti-retaliation policy in sufficient detail to be able to train employees in the contents of the policy and the procedures for reporting sexual harassment. Human Resources will likely have included a briefing on sexual harassment in the new-employee orientation, and there will likewise ordinarily be printed guidelines in both the employee handbook and the personnel policy manual.

It is essential that all employees know the process for reporting sexual harassment and be aware of the processes by which any charges of such behavior are investigated. Most organizations' reporting practices call for a complaining employee to address the problem with the immediate supervisor or manager. There are alternative procedures for complaining of harassment directly to Human Resources or to another point in the organization should an employee's immediate manager or supervisor be the subject of the complaint.

Sexually harassing behavior, although presently not nearly as prevalent as it was in the years before anti-discrimination legislation, remains a major concern throughout business and industry. It should remain a key concern of every department manager in the health care organization, and every manager would be well advised to maintain a zero-tolerance position where sexual harassment is concerned.

VIOLENCE

Violence in the workplace is often the result of stress; it frequently occurs when an individual becomes stressed to what for him or her is an unbearable level. When stress becomes unbearable some people become ill, some break down, some walk away from the situation—and some become violent. Violence is similar to other forms of human behavior in that it is action in response to a condition, need, or demand.

Every organizational change that alters expectations held by employees becomes fertile territory for chronic anger. Chronic anger can lead to diminished productivity, reduced quality, increased fatigue, burnout, depression, and violence. One in every six violent crimes occurs in the workplace. Whereas motor vehicle accidents are the leading cause of death for working men, murder is the leading cause of death for working women.

In the category of nonfatal assaults, the highest risk areas are the retail trades (grocery stores and eating and drinking establishments) and the service area (hospitals, nursing homes, and social services agencies). In the late 1990s it was determined that almost two-thirds of nonfatal assaults occurred in hospitals, nursing homes, and residential care facilities, with most cases involving patients assaulting nurses.[2] As with other potential sources of trouble, the department manager's best approach to workplace violence is awareness and prevention.

There is no consistent profile describing a person who commits violent acts in the workplace, but violence may be perpetrated by someone who:

- Is experiencing family problems, including, perhaps, a history of abuse
- Has problems stemming from substance abuse (alcohol or drugs)
- Has a history of violence

- Is a known aggressive personality
- Is experiencing certain mental conditions (e.g., depression)
- Possesses a poor self-image or low self-esteem.

There are no conclusive answers regarding why people commit violent acts, but the reasons behind workplace violence have been known to include:

- The inability to cope with what is perceived as an unbearable level of stress
- Drug reactions
- Problems involving job, money, or family
- Reaction to the loss of employment
- Reaction to the loss of a relationship
- Frustration with long waits or with what may be perceived as rude or indifferent treatment
- Confusion or fear
- Perceived violation of privacy.

Alert though we may be to the possibility of violence, we can never tell for certain who may resort to violence. However, a manager can take some steps to prevent violence:

- Treat everyone—employees, patients, visitors, and others—with respect and consideration.
- Keep all objects that could be used as weapons stored out of the reach of patients and visitors.
- Take threats seriously, reporting them immediately and through proper channels.
- Know your organization's security procedures, alarms, and warning codes.

Be extra alert to the possibility of violence if a person:

- Appears to be under the influence of alcohol or drugs
- Appears to have been in a fight
- Is brought into the facility by the police
- Is already being restrained.

Visible indicators of potential violence include:

- Obvious possession of a weapon
- Nervousness or abrupt movements
- Extreme restlessness, pacing, and obvious agitation
- Hitting walls, objects, etc.; breaking things.

When observing an individual who appears to be on the edge of losing control:

- Notify other staff and call the security department.
- Stay alert but remain calm.
- Maintain a safe distance, give the person plenty of space, and do not turn your back; do not *under any circumstances* touch the person.
- Keep obstacles between you and the individual.
- Be certain you have a way out—do not find yourself in a dead-end corridor or a corner.
- Listen; do not display anger or defensiveness and do not argue; speak slowly and quietly.

Some departments, for example the emergency room, are more likely sites of violence than others, but violence is possible anywhere in the facility. Therefore, each department's staff should have some orientation in how to deal with violent behavior. If violence does occur:

- Protect yourself to the extent necessary.
- Sound the alarm or call the appropriate code.
- Help remove others from the vicinity, if necessary.
- Do not try to disarm or restrain the person yourself.
- Give the individual what he or she is demanding, if possible.

EMPLOYEE PARTICIPATION AND INVOLVEMENT

Employee participation and involvement can often head off potential problems. However, participative management is not a program with a beginning and an end. The primary danger of formal "programs" with names and steering committees and such is that they come to be seen as something that will be here for a certain time and then gone.

Employee participation at any level—although here we are speaking primarily of participation at department level—requires management commitment. It is necessary to let employees know that you genuinely want and value their input, and also to let them know how to get their ideas into your hands. Eliciting participation requires that you listen to employees, and it requires that you be visible and available, out among the employees. The more employees feel that you are interested in what they do, the more they feel respected, challenged, and constructively utilized, the less likely they are to be troublesome.

Some few employees will want to do no more than what they are told, put in their hours, and go home. The majority of employees, however, would rather be challenged than not, would rather be interested than bored, and would rather feel that they are accomplishing something and not just simply putting in their time.

A great many people are capable of managing their own work if they are provided with the proper supportive environment and given the opportunity to perform. The manager had best never forget that nobody knows the inner detailed workings of a job better than the person who does it every day, and it is this source of knowledge that the manager should seek to tap through genuine participation.

A great many of the problems that a department manager faces occur at ground level, where the daily work is done, where hands-on care is delivered to the patients. Because of most rank-and-file employees' closeness to where so many of the problems occur, it only makes sense to have them participate in determining how improvements might be made and how problems might be solved. Generally, the higher a decision goes above the level it affects, the more likely that it will be wrong, so it makes extremely good sense to keep decision-making as close to the level of the problem as possible. Business executive and author Robert Townsend claimed that all decisions should be made as low as possible in the organizations, pointing out that "The Charge of the Light Brigade was ordered by an officer who wasn't there looking at the territory."[3]

The primary factor in the eventual success of employee involvement is supportive managerial behavior. The manager must be able to empower employees, not necessarily to always get them to develop the solutions or make the decisions but to understand how they influence processes and how they will contribute to decision-making.

The path to effective employee involvement requires a gradual transition; as mutual trust develops between manager and employees, each becomes more willing to help the other succeed. The organization or department that can achieve effective employee participation will usually experience significant increases in productivity and noticeable decreases in employee problems. Interested, stimulated, and challenged employees represent the best possible means of preventing problems in the department.

COUNSELING

Counseling is appropriate for addressing problems and potential problems at their early stages to keep them from becoming larger problems. Sometimes counseling simply involves the manager providing generalized guidance and work-related advice. Overall, counseling may be employed to:

- Catch problems in the early stages and attempt to head them off or fix them early
- Shore up weaknesses in employee performance and provide on-going guidance (sometimes called "coaching")
- Enable the manager to recommend developmental activities to the employee
- Generally improve communication between the manager and the employee.

It is always advisable to counsel an employee when a problem appears to be developing, rather than let the employee continue in an undesirable direction until disciplinary action or other corrective action is required. A need for counseling may be signaled by a number of circumstances, foremost among which are:

- A noticeable decline in an individual's performance or a person's failure to continue meeting job standards. A decline in performance, especially in an employee who has performed well for an extended period, often indicates a personal problem. A counseling session can afford the employee the opportunity to talk if he or she so desires, and thus the opportunity for the manager to make an appropriate referral.

- Violations of policies or work rules. As noted, it makes little sense to allow an employee to continue on a path toward disciplinary action when a friendly one-to-one counseling session may be able to head off further trouble.
- Changes in an individual relative to the job, for example, an employee who formerly seemed content who has become a chronic complainer, or an employee who seems to have lost motivation and no longer shows interest in the job.
- Deterioration of interpersonal relationships, for instance, an employee who formerly got along well with others who now is experiencing conflict with others.
- Complaints from patients, visitors, or other staff about an employee, especially regarding rude or inappropriate behavior on the part of an employee from whom these actions are contrary to past behavior.

For some managers, counseling may loom fully as frightening as public speaking, and it is certainly subject to the same general advice that can be applied to public speaking: it requires preparation and practice. Like speaking, the more one does it the more comfortable one becomes with it. Common obstacles to effective counseling include:

- The manager's perceived lack of counseling skills. However, this should not be considered a significant obstacle. Counseling is little different from interviewing, and as many managers have discovered, interviewing becomes easier as the interviewer grows more confident with experience.
- Time pressures. It often seems that there is never enough time to do all that should be done, and something like counseling, which often seems to have no immediate priority attached to it, is readily postponed, sometimes until it is forgotten.
- Friendships. Perhaps the manager was formerly an employee in the same department and must now manage the work of friends and long-time colleagues. Counseling friends is not much easier than disciplining friends, and some managers shy away from both activities.
- Deference to longevity or seniority. Some managers, especially those younger or newer to their positions, may avoid speaking

up to employees who have been involved in the same kind of work much longer than they have.

- Fear of legal problems. Recent years have given most managers good reason to be wary of making mistakes that can get the organization into legal trouble, and some see remaining silent as the only way to completely avoid the chance of making such mistakes. Silence, however, can be fully as risky as speech, so avoidance may not be the safest approach legally.

To provide effective counseling:

- Be knowledgeable and credible. Know what you are talking about. If you are hesitant to counsel because of a lack of knowledge, investigate the problem, research the subject, and ask Human Resources for guidance.
- Keep your consoling consistent from person to person. Just as you would in addressing any of the corrective processes, make certain that what applies to one can apply equally to all others who are similarly situated.
- Stay specific, never generalize. As in delivering criticism or addressing negatives of any nature, always address specific problems, incidents, complaints, etc.
- Be timely. As with delaying disciplinary action, delaying counseling until a later time dilutes the message and diminishes its impact.
- Be alert for employee defensiveness, and do not argue. Some employees will take any effort at counseling as direct criticism and will immediately become defensive. Should this occur, hear the employee out and avoid contradicting the person if possible.
- Be as positive as possible. Counseling may indeed contain elements of criticism, but surely there is something about the person that will permit you to cast a positive light on much of the discussion.
- Listen, really listen. In counseling you may be required to speak more than in, say, selection interviewing or appraisal interviewing, but when the employee is speaking provide your undivided attention and tune in to what is really being said.

The department manager needs to remember at all times that his or her primary interest concerning employee behavior should be in the *results* of behavior, never the causes. In counseling, never attempt to infer the cause of behavior, and do not attempt to pry for it. Focus on the results of behavior and on getting that behavior corrected, but steer clear of the employee's personal life.

Document each counseling session briefly and informally, making note of employee name, date, and nature of the discussion. Try to capture the essence of the discussion anecdotally and objectively. This documentation need not be considered a permanent record, but it should be retained for a period of time in the event the problem recurs.

Discussion Points

1. Explain why our primary interest should be the *results* of employee behavior. Shouldn't we be trying to eliminate *causes*?
2. Describe in detail at least one employment-related area of activity in which there is a continuing conflict between the needs of the health care organization and the privacy rights of the individual.
3. Explain how a department manager might go about preventing excessive absenteeism among employees.
4. Describe in some detail a hypothetical scenario in which you believe the polygraph testing of an employee would be legal.
5. Explain why it is advisable to maintain documentation having a bearing on employee health issues separate from the regular personnel file.
6. Describe the circumstances under which a department manager may be granted access to the personnel files of employees of other departments.
7. Discuss why employee involvement is frequently recommended as a strategy for problem prevention.
8. Discuss why a manager should take the time to counsel an employee when a disciplinary problem appears in the making. Explain why the manager shouldn't wait until definitive disciplinary action is permissible under the organization's policies.

9. Describe two hypothetical actions concerning an employee's financial status that probably cannot legally be taken because of the passage of the Fair Credit Reporting Act.
10. Explain why it is necessary to obtain an employee's written permission before releasing any information concerning that employee to an interest external to the organization. Specify when such information may be released without employee permission.

NOTES

[1]Williams Petrocelli, *Low Profile—How to Avoid the Privacy Invader* (New York: McGraw-Hill Book Company, 1981), p. 112.

[2]"Preventing Violence in the Workplace," Group Insurance Agency, Inc., Healthcare Association of New York State, Albany, NY, May 9, 1997.

[3]Robert Townsend, *Up the Organization: How to Stop the Corporation from Stifling People and Strangling Profits* (New York: Fawcett World Library, 1971), p. 27.

CHAPTER 12

Employee Documentation: Shoulds and Should-Nots for the Manager

This chapter—

- Differentiates between formal documentation (which results from compliance with laws and regulations) and informal documentation (which is not legally required but is helpful in running an organization)
- Reviews the legal implications of employment documentation
- Addresses the Human Resources role in maintaining and safeguarding personnel files
- Outlines the department manager's responsibilities relating to employment documentation
- Advises the department manager with regard to creating and maintaining anecdotal note files concerning employees
- Stresses the importance of complete, properly executed, and properly retained documentation.

PAPER REMAINS IMPORTANT

It may seem as though a large and ever-increasing percentage of the civilized world is kept running according to what appears on a computer screen or is stored on a hard drive or disk. Despite the encroachment of electronic technology, however, paper still dominates in many respects. Even a great deal of what is captured on a computer is converted to printed form for a number of important uses.

Much documentation is intended as simple record-keeping, ensuring that certain documents are available for reference if need be and for various other ordinary business purposes. However, since the introduction of major civil rights legislation in the 1960s, an increasing amount of documentation has been created and maintained largely as protection against legal challenges.

The emphasis of this chapter is on various forms of employment documentation. Medical documentation will not be addressed here, although we should be aware that medical documentation is a relevant concern for managers of clinical activities. In a number of ways medical documentation has been regularly receiving most of the attention it deserves, but employment documentation has not received nearly enough conscientious attention.

Two general classes of employment documentation will be examined:

- Formal documentation, which results primarily from adherence to laws or regulatory requirements, such as the majority of the items found in an employee's personnel file
- Informal documentation, which is not required by law or regulation but deemed helpful in running an organization, such as internal reports, statistics, meeting minutes, and anecdotal notes.

Documentation can be troublesome for the department manager in two ways: (1) when we do not have it and it appears never to have existed, and (2) when it exists but is weak, inaccurate, or incomplete.

LEGAL IMPLICATIONS OF EMPLOYMENT DOCUMENTATION

Every piece of paper ever generated concerning an employee is a potential key in turning a legal complaint for or against the organization or the manager. Evidence of discrimination or the absence of that evidence is often inferred from what is found in documentation relating to employees. The most common kind of discrimination charges involves differential treatment, specifically, alleged violations of Title VII of the Civil Rights Act of 1964, which requires that all individuals be treated equally concerning terms and conditions of employment. The next most common kind of discrimination charges involves allegations of disparate impact, which result from job requirements or actions of the employer that have a discriminatory effect on a protected group. When either type of charge is under examination, documentation concerning all affected employees is brought into the process.

Employment documentation is always important in addressing charges of discrimination. If the required documentation cannot be produced, often the worst is assumed.

Any documentation related in any way to a person's employment can be called upon in a legal action. Under a legal order known as a *notice to produce*, an organization can be required to produce for copying and inspection any documents that may be possibly or even remotely related to the charge. The notice to produce can ask for a considerable variety of material, including:

- The personnel files of persons involved in the action. This can be far-reaching, calling for a great many personnel files. For example, in a particular action in which three employees charged a history of discriminatory behavior that followed them from their former departments to their present situation, the personnel files of all employees in all affected departments were requested ("demanded" might be a better word when it comes to these kinds of "requests"). This amounted to nearly 100 personnel files.
- The organization's personnel policy and procedure manual, including all policies applicable to the complaining employees' employment. Initially this request may seem readily satisfied by handing a copy of the manual over to plaintiff's legal counsel. At times it can be precisely that easy, but it can also become complicated because personnel polices may be revised periodically as circumstances change. For example, consider a particular action that involved alleged discriminatory acts committed over a period of two to three years. Several policies that could conceivably have had a bearing on the complaint had been revised during the period, so the notice to produce demanded not only the policy manual but each policy in each of its various forms dating back to before the alleged discrimination began. (The lesson in this for the Human Resources department is to maintain a documented revision trail for all policies in the manual.)
- The organization's employee handbook, and its revision history if pertinent to the time period of the alleged discrimination.
- Copies of all other work rules, regulations, etc., that the complaining employees are alleged by the employer to have broken,

and all documentation related in any way to the handling of such allegations.

- Copies of all job postings and employment advertisements relevant to the departments of the complaining employees dating back to before the alleged discrimination began.
- Copies of any informal files the department manager has maintained concerning the complaining employees.

More information concerning the legal implications of employment documentation will be presented in Chapter 14, See You in Court: Involvement in Legal Action. Suffice it to say at this point that any information that cannot legally be the basis for a personnel decision should never enter an employee's personnel file and should never be retained in a manager's anecdotal files.

RECORD RETENTION

Some records are retained because common sense suggests that legitimate needs to retrieve the information they contain may arise sometime in the future. Certain records are retained because external requirements dictate their retention. All federal laws that address aspects of the employment relationship include record retention requirements. For the most part, retention is a continuing responsibility of Human Resources.

Most regulatory agencies that administer employment legislation specify the minimum length of time that pertinent records must be retained. Most such specified retention periods are different from each other. For example:

- Under the Fair Labor Standards Act, payroll records and supporting information (time cards, times sheets, etc.) must be retained for three years, and other related information (job evaluations, merit system descriptions and records, payroll deduction records, etc.) must be retained for two years.
- Under the Age Discrimination in Employment Act, all employment-related records must be retained for one year (consistent with the provision that a charge of discrimination under ADEA must be filed within one year of the alleged act of discrimination).
- The Occupational Safety and Health Administration requires that all records of employee injury or illness be retained for five years.

- Under Title VII of the Civil Rights Act of 1964, all records of personnel transactions must be retained for at least six months, unless charges are filed, in which instances the records must be retained until after final disposition of the charges.

The Joint Commission on the Accreditation of Healthcare Organizations (JCAHO) requires that a number of classes of documentation be retained so they can be reviewed during periodic accreditation surveys, including all:

- Documents that demonstrate compliance with federal laws
- Licenses held by the organization and its individual personnel
- Records of employee training
- Detailed records of safety practices
- Policies and procedures
- Job descriptions
- Employee performance appraisals.

In its periodic surveys, the health department of the state in which the organization is located may also look for much the same documentation that JCAHO requires. In addition, states having right-to-know laws concerning toxic substances will be interested in those particular records.

Hazardous material and toxic substances present some of the most rigid record-retention requirements found in any businesses. Under the Occupational Safety and Health Act, records of any personal or environmental monitoring of exposure to hazardous materials must be retained for 30 years. The 30-year requirements also hold for records retained in response to the Toxic Substances Control Act administered by the Environmental Protection Agency. Within New York State, records of exposure retained in response to the New York State Right-to-Know Law must be kept for 40 years.

The threshold for retaining most employment documentation is six years, which is also the statutory limit for filing most employment-related charges arising from consideration of Title VII of the Civil Rights Act of 1964.

There is such a mix of required retention periods, conceivably ranging from 6 months to 40 years, that many organizations simply assume that they will be retaining all personnel files permanently. Employees come and go, generating files that become inactive. Some employees who remain for many years generate thick files over the course of their employment. All these files can accrue to considerable volume over the course of a few years, so Human Resources is often faced with a record-retention challenge.

Personnel files of employees who have moved on to other employment must often be accessed in responding to reference requests and other legitimate external requests for information concerning past employees, and to bring forward the past records of former employees who return. Therefore, files of past employees, at least of those who have left within the most recent few years, must be accessible. It is generally true that the older the file the less likely it is to be called for, so a Human Resources approach to the retention of personnel files will often be to keep the newest records most accessible. Many HR departments do not have the luxury of unlimited record storage space, so microfilming older personnel records has become a fairly common practice.

For example, before deciding to microfilm personnel records, one mid-sized hospital first conducted a detailed study to develop a retrieval profile based on how likely a record was to be accessed during each year that it aged. This profile was compared with the amount of space the hospital could devote to hard-copy personnel records. A plan was developed under which eight years of hard-copy records of past employees were retained (in reverse chronological order by year), and everything older was committed to microfilm. At the end of each year the older year of hard-copy records was then committed to microfilm, so that the HR department always had access to at least eight years but never more than nine years of hard copies, with everything older on microfilm.

HUMAN RESOURCES AND THE PERSONNEL FILE

Employee documentation is primarily the responsibility of the Human Resources department, so it falls to HR to ensure that everything that must be retained in the personnel file is in fact there and complete. The department manager's role in supporting the personnel file consists primarily of ensuring that departmental inputs to the personnel file get to Human Resources properly completed and in a timely fashion. Foremost among the documents coming from the department manager are performance appraisals and disciplinary actions, plus certain routine employee information that may pass through the manager, such as changes of address for employees.

The department manager should expect to hear from Human Resources if certain documentation is not forthcoming. Performance appraisals and disciplinary actions are most likely to be the subjects of such follow-up. Depending on how the organization keeps track of current licensure, Human Resources may also look to the department managers to ensure that licensed caregivers renew their licenses in a timely fashion and submit copies for their personnel files or a central license repository.

Personnel policies may include a policy governing the "life" of disciplinary actions. For example, there may be a policy stating that a written warning in an employee's file will be considered "expired" if some period of time—perhaps 18 or 24 months—passes without subsequent related infractions. If this is a practice, Human Resources will monitor the age of warnings and invalidate them as the proper time elapses. The HR staff will not necessarily go through all personnel files to remove expired warnings, but when outdated warnings are encountered as files are reviewed or material is filed, they will be removed (usually to an inactive file).

The Human Resources department will control access to personnel files. Internal access to personnel files will ordinarily be limited to:

- Certain employees of Human Resources (some may have no need to access personnel files)
- An employee's immediate chain of command (the employee's manager, that manager's manager, etc.)
- The organization's legal counsel (in addressing specific questions)
- Interested managers reviewing records to assess potential transfer candidates
- Employees exercising the right to review their own personnel files (usually under HR supervision, with a prohibition against removing any documents).

Access to a personnel file (or a portion thereof) by interests external to the organization is strictly limited to:

- Documents covered by a release signed by the affected employee extending permission to release specific information (for example, in answering reference requests or applying for a mortgage loan)
- Documents or personnel files that must be released in response to a legal subpoena or court order.

Guidelines for addressing the confidentiality of employee records are presented in Exhibit 12-1. These guidelines are based on principles developed in 1973 by a U.S. Department of Health, Education, and Welfare task force.

THE DEPARTMENT MANAGER'S RESPONSIBILITIES

The department manager has responsibility related to employee documentation in several specific areas.

Job Descriptions

Too often the current status of a job description—and sometimes, in fact, the very existence of a job description—is given no thought until the document is needed. It is usually not until a job description is needed that someone realizes that it is missing or sadly out of date—for example, when HR is preparing to recruit and would like to place an advertisement. Without a complete, up-to-date job description, chances are that HR cannot accurately describe the job for recruiting purposes.

The department manager and Human Resources are often required to work together on job descriptions. Usually the content will come from the manager, and HR will provide the format and some of the "boilerplate" items that are part of most job descriptions. Revising

---

Exhibit 12-1   Guidelines for Confidentiality of Employee Information

- Employees must know of the existence of all systems of retaining personal information; no such systems should be kept secret from employees.
- There must be a procedure for individuals to determine what information exists about them and how it is to be used.
- Personal information obtained for one purpose cannot be used for other purposes without the consent of the individual to whom the information pertains.
- There must be a process by which individuals are able to correct or amend records of personal information pertaining to them.
- Any organization that creates, maintains, and uses or disseminates identifiable personal information must ensure the reliability of the information for the intended use and must take steps to prevent the misuse of the information.

and updating a job description for an existing position should, if at all possible, include the employee presently doing the job. Certainly employees should be involved in an annual review and update of their job descriptions.

A word of caution concerning job descriptions: Try to avoid having different versions of the same job description in circulation. Often when a job description is updated, there are various copies "out there" that do not necessarily get collected and destroyed. It is best to keep track of who has copies of a particular job description, and at update time see that these are all gathered and replaced. If in doubt about whether a given job description is current, have Human Resources check it against the master job description file (which most HR departments maintain) to ensure that you have the current version.

Employee Handbook

If the organization has an employee handbook, the department manager should be conversant with its contents for two reasons: (1) for personal knowledge and use, since the manager is also an employee; and (2) to answer employees' questions to some reasonable extent. As manager you do not need to know the handbook so well that you can handle every related question without looking up anything, but you ought to be able to handle general questions about the handbook's contents and also know how and where to obtain clarification regarding any of the handbook's contents.

Also, make certain that all employees in the department have the *current* handbook. Employee handbooks are not revised as often as policy and procedure manuals, but new editions are usually issued every few years. When the handbook is reissued and circulated to all employees, make certain that each employee not only receives one but also executes and submits a receipt acknowledging that he or she has received *and read* the handbook. Handbooks include work rules as well as general information about the organization, and may even include information concerning key personnel policies. A signed handbook receipt, made part of an employee's personnel files, is retained as evidence that the employee has received and reviewed the handbook. This can be extremely important to the organization should an employee attempt to deny knowledge of a particular rule or policy as an excuse for a rule violation.

Policy and Procedure Manuals

The organization's personnel policy and procedure manual is ordinarily issued by Human Resources, and most policies are prepared by HR either directly or based on other organizational input and distributed by HR. In most organizations every department will have a copy of the manual; some larger departments may have multiple copies.

Advice to the department manager, or whoever is the "keeper" of the department's policy and procedure manual: File updates as they are received—do not let them accumulate. There will always come a time when quick reference to a specific policy is required, and if the manual has not been kept up to date it will not be possible to know whether a given policy is current or not. It is a great temptation to let policy and procedure updates drift to the bottom of the in-basket, to be saved for a "better time" to file them away. There is usually no better time than when they are received, and a manual that has been allowed to go out of date can be useless if not damaging if a wrong reference is taken as applicable.

Do not consider the department policy and procedure manual to be a "manager's" book, kept in your office for your exclusive use. Keep the policy and procedure manual out where employees can get at it and make reference to it when they need to, without having to ask for it. If the manual is retained in someone's office and cannot be readily accessed, employees are left feeling that it is kept from them and that there is something "secret" about it. Personnel policies are there for all employees, and all employees deserve equal access to the manual.

Giving Out Employee Information

As department manager you may occasionally receive both internal and external requests for information about particular employees. Should you receive requests for employee information from outside of the organization, do not respond. Refer the requester to the appropriate point in the organization, usually Human Resources. The HR position concerning external release of employee information should be the entire organization's position on this matter: Nothing about an employee gets released to the outside without the employee's signed consent or a legal order (subpoena, court order, etc.).

Concerning requests from within the organization—for example, from another manager who asks you about the performance of an employee who is being considered as a transfer candidate—respond strictly on a need-to-know basis. When responding, keep opinion and subjective assessments out of the transaction; provide only objective information that can be supported by an official record (e.g., performance appraisal, attendance records).

DEPARTMENT MANAGER'S EMPLOYEE FILES

The department manager will have occasion to keep certain records, both formal and informal, concerning each employee. Employee records maintained in the department need not be considered permanent; there is but one permanent record of employment, and that is the personnel file maintained by Human Resources. However, the files maintained by the manager should not be approached carelessly or even casually. The manager may believe that whatever files he or she maintains separately are personal property, never to be seen by others. This is a dangerous assumption, as the occasional manager has discovered; under certain circumstances these files could be made public (see Chapter 14, See You in Court: Involvement in Legal Action).

Regardless of how much or how little there may be to file concerning any particular employee, it is always best to maintain a file folder for each employee. You should avoid placing yourself in a situation in which it could be claimed that you kept files on some employees and not on others, the implication being that you selectively "watched" some employees while others were allowed to go their own way.

Your file for each employee will ordinarily include:

- Copies of the employee's most recent one or two performance appraisals (no need to keep many years' worth of appraisals, since these are always available in the personnel file in HR).
- Notes reminding yourself of items, both positive and negative as appropriate, to include in the employee's next performance appraisal.
- Copies of warnings, reprimands, or other disciplinary information concerning the employee. (Depending on the particular disciplinary system, a record of oral warning may remain with the manager instead of going to Human Resources; it would be forwarded to HR along with a written warning for a similar subsequent offense.)
- Accurate records of any performance improvement activities undertaken, including all indications of follow-up and problem resolution.

- Copies of complaints or compliments received concerning the employee (which should have been discussed with the employee at the time they were received).
- Notes of counseling sessions held with the employee.
- Any other information relevant to the individual's employment or performance in the department that is not customarily included in the formal documentation required of a personnel file.

It is essential that everything the manager writes for the employee's departmental file be expressed in accurate, objective language without name-calling or insupportable opinions. Be forever mindful of the possibility of external scrutiny of your records, always thinking: What would it sound like if this were made public?

Periodically clean out your employee files. For example, when performance appraisal time comes and goes, purge the notes that were meant to remind you of items to address in the appraisal. Get rid of old counseling notes if the problems prompting the counseling have not recurred for a year or two.

Sometimes your employee files can grow to encompass a considerable amount of paper, most of which will be useless to anyone. You can safely clean out your employee files at any time, with a single exception: Should a legal action begin and the organization be in receipt of a legal *notice to produce* that asks for these files, it is a law violation to destroy any related records once the notice is received. Routine cleanout when no legal trouble is looming is fine; should something be legally requested later, it cannot be produced if it does not exist.

DO THE PAPERWORK

Documentation is one of those tasks that frequently get put off. Unfortunately, documentation left until there is more time to do it often does not get done thoroughly or perhaps does not get done at all. Documentation should be timely. Even in the immediate presence of "too much to do" and other pressures on the manager, it is best to address documentation right away because that is when facts are freshest in one's mind and thus when the most accurate documentation is created.

Many problems occur after the fact because of missing or incomplete documentation. Instances of incomplete documentation are common in every organization—forms not completely filled out, forms not signed, information entered partially or illegibly. And there is one nagging problem that surfaces time and again with documentation that could be avoided completely if we all remembered one incredibly simple rule: Every time one prepares to put words on paper in any format, whether formal or informal, the very first step to take is—*put the date on the page.* This simple act would solve a great many subsequent problems with documentation.

Discussion Points

1. Describe the full implications of the statement: "If it isn't in the personnel file, it never happened."
2. Discuss why the majority of health care organizations have adopted the practice of permanently retaining the personnel files of past employees. Enumerate the particular kinds of records that have been largely responsible for the indefinite retention of personnel records.
3. Discuss why it should be the organization's practice to retain all documentation that must legally be retained, but to periodically clean out and dispose of unneeded documentation.
4. Specify under what circumstances an employee might be permitted to add an item to or remove an item from his or her personnel file.
5. Identify the most frequently occurring problems associated with the creation and retention of business documentation. How can these be addressed?
6. Explain why it should it be considered necessary for the department manager to keep the organization's personnel policy and procedure manual readily available to employees. Consider whether each person's employee handbook is sufficient.
7. You are a department manager. You receive a written request for reference information concerning a past employee. It is addressed to you personally, and it includes the former employee's written permission to release information. Explain how you should handle this request, and why.
8. Discuss why the manager should always remain objective, factual, and nonjudgmental in maintaining private anecdotal

note files concerning employees when it is intended that no one but their author will ever see them.

9. Explain why a manager's anecdotal note files should be periodically purged of all but currently essential information.

10. Describe how and why some documentation can be more damaging to the organization in a legal matter by being missing and unattainable rather than readily available.

CHAPTER 13

Terminating Employees: Minimizing the Legal Risks

This chapter—

- Addresses the roles of Human Resources and the department manager in terminating employees, whether discharged for cause, dismissed for performance reasons, or laid off as a result of a reduction in force
- Describes the concept of constructive discharge
- Describes the conditions that have been contributing to mass terminations (layoffs) in health care
- Recommends steps to consider before deciding to lay off personnel
- Reviews various means of determining who goes and who remains in a layoff
- Reviews related dimensions of termination, including unemployment compensation and employee privacy
- Examines the potential effects on the survivors of a layoff and suggests how management can address these.

INDIVIDUAL TERMINATIONS

Throughout this book, we have made a distinction between *discharge* and *dismissal*. What we refer to as *discharged* is best equated with the age-old term *fired*; it occurs because of rule-breaking or policy violation. What we call *dismissal* is best characterized as *laid off*; it occurs for performance-related reasons such as failure to pass the probationary period or failure to meet the minimum standards of the job.

Discharge: Termination for Cause

Having to fire someone is the dread of many managers, even if the firing is completely deserved (and any such termination had better be completely deserved). Doing so is one of those few management tasks that are not easy to begin with and rarely get easier even with repetition. In fact, firing someone should never be easy; there should always be an emotional price to pay for severing someone from his or her livelihood, regardless of the reason. If a manager can coldly and unfeelingly discharge an employee, perhaps that manager should not be a manager.

For this discussion, it is assumed that the department manager has worked with the Human Resources department, that HR and the manager are in agreement on the termination, and that all required information is in place (see the discussion of progressive disciplinary processes in Chapter 9, The Health Care Manager and Employee Problems).

The "best" involuntary terminations from the employer's point of view, that is, those terminations that occur with least risk to the organizations, are those for which:

- Good cause is evident
- The organization closely followed its own policies
- The organization can demonstrate, should the question be pertinent, that the employee was given every reasonable opportunity to correct the offending behavior.

It is always essential to ensure that (1) the organization's policies have been followed in terms of the progressive disciplinary steps applicable to the specific problem, and (2) all proper documentation is complete and in place. Overall, the most important dimension of termination for cause is making certain that all pertinent policies and processes are followed.

Despite the best efforts of department management and Human Resources, however, the organization can sometimes be trapped by unexpected circumstances. For example, in years past certain written passages in employee handbooks—such as one saying that an employee who passes probation becomes a "permanent" employee—have been interpreted as constituting "contracts" of employment and used to protest discharge. As such problems are encountered, they are corrected—the formerly "permanent" employee becomes a "regular" employee in the handbook—and after the system has been tested a few times and the weak spots have been identified, it can be expected to function as intended.

The department manager should be prepared for the possibility that any member of what is defined as a "protected class" under Equal Employment Opportunity may claim discrimination in being discharged. Regardless of the real reasons for such termination, the situation often immediately becomes complicated with a charge such as "I was let go because of my _____" (race, color, creed, gender, age, disability, religion, etc.).

No department manager or Human Resources representative wants to become involved in a wrongful termination lawsuit. These are usually frustrating, costly, and time-consuming exercises that do not necessarily resolve themselves fairly (plaintiffs' attorneys strongly seek jury trials for employment cases because juries tend to side with the individual as opposed to the organization).

Regardless of the care that goes into a discharge, there is always the risk of an unlawful discharge claim. Anyone can file a charge with the Equal Employment Opportunity Commission or the state division of human rights, and anyone who can secure the services of an attorney can sue. The organization's best protections are:

- Fair personnel policies, applied consistently
- A fair performance appraisal system
- Complete and available documentation
- Clear evidence of wrongdoing.

Dismissal: Inability to Meet Job Standards

Dismissal is related to performance, and the individual is not considered at fault as is in discharge, where the individual committed a violation or infraction. Since no rule is broken and no policy is violated, dismissal for inability to meet the standards of the job or for failure to pass the probationary period is treated more as a layoff than a discharge. The distinction becomes important when we consider what often comes *after* termination, specifically an application for unemployment compensation. One who is discharged—that is, fired for cause—is considered ineligible for unemployment compensation, while one who is dismissed—that is, laid off—is assumed to be eligible for unemployment compensation.

Whether or not the organization internally makes the distinction between these two kinds of involuntary separation, the difference in external recourse will distinguish between the two. The majority of employees who are involuntarily separated apply for unemployment benefits regardless of the circumstances under which they were let go. If many who were legitimately discharged apply anyway because they feel they have nothing to lose by doing so, some find their assumption was correct. Discharged employees are frequently granted unemployment compensation even if they have been discharged for cause.

One purpose of recommending an organizational distinction between discharge and dismissal is to suggest that an organization should not attempt to deny unemployment benefits to someone whose only shortcoming (not transgression, because it did not involve a rule or policy violation) was the inability to perform to the standards of the job.

Constructive Discharge

Occasionally we find a manager who seems to believe that the most effective way of getting rid of an under-producing or uncooperative employee is simply to keep piling on the work until the person finally quits. After all, the manager might reason, someone who resigns voluntarily is not eligible for unemployment compensation, and we have solved a problem without having to openly fire an employee. However, there is a significant risk in getting rid of an employee in this fashion.

The concept of *constructive discharge* comes into consideration when an ex-employee registers a legal complaint in which it is alleged that the organization, usually as represented by one of its managers, made life so difficult and unbearable that the individual had to resign or experience physical illness or emotional damage by remaining. A resignation that is not strictly voluntary, in the sense that it is in effect forced by extreme or intolerable conditions or treatment, may be considered a constructive discharge.

A potential constructive discharge is the condition that pertains when an individual who is approaching termination for cause is allowed to resign in lieu of discharge. Occasionally well-intended management will even suggest that an individual be allowed to resign "for the record" in lieu of discharge, perhaps thinking it is better for the individual to avoid having an involuntary termination in the personnel record. However, this sets up the organization for a claim of constructive discharge—"I had to resign because I was going to be fired if I didn't." It is far safer for the organization, and thus for the department manager, to follow through with discharge, well documented of course, if that is what organizational policy calls for.

REDUCTIONS IN FORCE

It is difficult to pick up any publication that addresses present-day health care issues without seeing something about health care costs. For some time, the amounts that the third-party payers have been reimbursing the providers of care have been shrinking or have been constrained from growing at the rate that the cost of delivering care is growing. Pressures on providers continue to mount, as government and the public push the industry to contain or reduce costs while maintaining or improving quality and continually incorporating technological advances in medical care. The health care industry is under constant pressure to do more with less, and since as much as two-thirds of a hospital's cost is people, substantial cuts in reimbursement inevitably affect people.

The ever-changing economics of health care lead in significant part to the elimination of health care jobs.

Reengineering

Health care organizations entered into reengineering a few years after it peaked in manufacturing. We can describe reengineering as: *The systematic redesign of a business's core processes, starting with desired outcomes and establishing the most efficient possible processes to achieve those outcomes."* Reengineering has also been referred to by variety of other names, including downsizing, rightsizing, reorganizing, repositioning, revitalizing, and modernizing. To a great many employees, reengineering and all of these synonymous processes have one single significant result: job loss. Whichever term is used, however it happens to be used, and no matter how carefully it is used, its mere mention in any official organizational context immediately alerts employees to the likelihood of layoffs. Consider: "Reengineering—so popular among hospital executives just a few years ago—is a double-edged word: On one hand, rethinking the flow of work can save money, increase margins, and keep a struggling hospital afloat. On the other hand, reengineering almost always leads to the layoffs, increased outsourcings, and unit closings that employees feared from the start."[1]

Many fearful employees have good reason to equate reengineering with downsizing: Some 81 percent of reengineered hospitals have trimmed their staffs through layoffs or attrition, and nearly half have laid off managers as well.[2]

Employee morale is the most severe Human Resources problem in the hospital sector, and the main cause of the morale problem is layoffs of hospital personnel. There seems to be no way to avoid the conclusion that reengineering equals jobs eliminated.

Mergers, Acquisitions, and Other Affiliations

Mergers, acquisitions, and other forms of affiliation have become a way of life in health care. Since these combinations are usually entered into in response to financial pressures, they usually mean the loss of jobs. Health care has seen essentially all possible forms of affiliation and combination, including the formation of multi-organizational health systems.

Systems often promote diversification and breadth of services. Not-for-profit systems are usually more diversified than for-profit systems; the for-profit systems more often tend to specialize, and they are far less likely to sustain a service that is not profitable. Not-for-profit systems are more likely to carry unprofitable services for the sake of remaining "full service" to the communities they serve.

There has been little evidence to suggest that hospitals belonging to multi-organizational systems are any more efficient than free-standing hospitals. In some parts of the country, systems and other alliances have been the salvation of endangered rural hospitals but usually at the cost of job loss in the rural communities.

Mergers frequently lead to the reduction of management positions as well as staff positions. Consider the merger of two small-town hospitals located not far from each other. The merger involved the combination of parallel departments of both institutions under single management; for example, where before there were two clinical laboratories with two managers, there was now a two-location laboratory department with a single manager. The result of this merger was about 12 fewer managers, with each remaining manager left with a greatly enlarged span of control.

The process of merger is usually considerably more difficult and more expensive than originally anticipated. Employees of one organization will usually fear absorption by the other organization and loss of identity. And this is more or less what happens; even a so-called merger of equals essentially results in one organization taking over the other.

Consolidation expenses can be high and can take an extremely long time to pay themselves back in lower operating costs and improved efficiency. Also, such organizational combinations can be highly disruptive to staff in a number of ways as possibly conflicting organizational cultures are forced to mix. The human side of merger or acquisition is usually not given sufficient attention; the emotional issues, those that can make or break a consolidation, usually take a distant second place to the financial issues.

If your organization is investigating the possibility of merger or affiliation, as department manager you may not be privy to much useful information, especially in the early stages. Yet as long as the word is out concerning the possibility, your employees will be uneasy. Maintain dialogue with your employees—listen to them, hear their concerns, keep them informed of what little you may know. Be honest about the possibilities—surely you want to avoid saying "Don't worry, it will never happen" just before a merger *does* happen—and keep contact open and do your best to get answers for your employees when you can.

Layoffs

Department management and Human Resources alike experience considerable stress when it becomes necessary to implement mass layoffs. When a layoff is impending, the organization should have planned sufficiently in advance to have first taken certain steps:

- Make all realistic non-labor savings.
- Eliminate the use of all temporary employees, whether hired by the organization or secured through temporary help agencies.
- Institute a hiring freeze. Stopping the influx of all but absolutely essential staff may provide time to consider internal reallocation of personnel.
- Close down most of the open positions, which can reduce the total number of positions without releasing people.
- Consider offering a voluntary termination incentive.
- Consider offering an early retirement incentive. (Specific individuals or groups cannot be targeted—to do so is discrimina-

tory—so there is always the risk that some key employees the organization would want to retain actually leave.)

Who Goes and Who Stays?

The department manager will probably be involved to some extent in determining who goes and who stays, although such decisions must proceed according to organizational guidelines that are ordinarily established by Administration and Human Resources with the guidance of legal counsel. Selection for layoff is most commonly accomplished by seniority, although this need not be so unless there is a union contract governing selection for layoff. Assessment mechanisms often consider a combination of factors that may include seniority, performance (as reflected by appraisals), attendance, and conduct (history of disciplinary actions). If the employees are represented by a union, chances are that the contract between the employer and the union will spell out, often in considerable detail, how employees are chosen for layoff.

Many organizations have discovered that seniority is both the fairest and safest means of determining who goes and who stays. Even using seniority alone, however, questions arise about how seniority is determined. It might be:

- Seniority in the organization
- Seniority in the department
- Seniority within a function or job class
- Seniority within function within department.

Related to seniority, or at least affecting how seniority is assessed, is the process of *bumping*. Bumping occurs when the job of an individual of greater seniority is eliminated, allowing that person to "bump" an individual of lesser seniority out of his or her position, and so on down the line until the individual of least seniority goes on layoff. Bumping can be simple or it can become extremely complex, depending on the rules in place.

Health care organizations in general, and hospitals in particular, often use considerable numbers of part-time employees. The official approach taken to selecting employees for layoff may include guidelines for the order of reduction based on work status. For example, a requirement may state that after temporary employees are released, next in line for reductions are regular part-time employees; that is, part-time employees may be released before regular full-time employees begin to be released.

Whatever combination of approaches and considerations the organization uses, however, the most important factor in how the guidelines are applied is *consistency*. Ideally the organization should have a personnel policy to govern staff reductions. This policy should be in place well before reductions ever become necessary; in many organizations, however, no policy is created until the need for reductions is close at hand. In some organizations it is likely that establishing such a policy simply has not occurred to anyone, given that the specter of layoffs has never before arisen; in others perhaps a layoff policy was overlooked either out of denial ("It will never happen here") or for fear that planning for a staff reduction could become a self-fulfilling prophecy.

Exhibit 13-1 is a sample reduction-in-force (RIF) policy illustrating how one hospital organization might have addressed most of the foregoing concerns.

Once a layoff plan is decided upon, Administration, Human Resources, and legal counsel need to assess the layoff plan carefully to ensure the absence of bias. If there is a discernible pattern among those marked for reduction—age, gender, race, etc.—charges of discrimination could arise. Some organizations have experienced problems, for example, with layoffs that involved a preponderance of older employees. An organization's intent may have been to reduce costs by removing higher-paid employees, but more than once it has been determined that since higher average pay correlates directly with more advanced age, the selection for layoff based on pay level was in fact age discrimination. All such possibilities need to be examined before a reduction plan can be considered workable.

In the process of a reduction the organization will be trying to become leaner while retaining the best employees. This may be difficult, however, when the more senior employees of a protected classification are dropped in preference to newer employees who possess critical skills.

The Timing of Layoffs

From the employee point of view, there is little if anything positive about a layoff, no matter what timing is involved. Consultants and

Exhibit 13-1 Model Policy and Procedure: Reduction in Force

Policy

The Hospital's employees are best served by continuous employment. However, there may be occasions when it is necessary to reduce staffing levels because of changing financial or operating circumstances. The objective of this policy is to provide a rational basis for the reduction of staffing levels in the event such adjustments are necessary.

Definitions

Department—a cost center or set of cost centers having common positions, functions, and duties reporting to the same manager.

Hospital seniority—one's uninterrupted service time as a full-time or part-time employee of the Hospital, adjusted for approved leaves of absence.

Department seniority—one's uninterrupted service time as a full-time or part-time employee of one's present department or unit, adjusted for approved leaves of absence.

Incumbent employee—an employee currently occupying an approved full-time or part-time position.

Qualified employee—one who possesses the stated qualifications for a specific position by virtue of education, experience, or both, and can either presently perform in that position or achieve standard performance within the normal introductory period.

Determination of Staff Reduction
A. Work Force Composition
1. Establishment of the size, composition, and distribution of the Hospital's work force remains a prerogative of management.
2. Before deciding that staff reduction is necessary, management will investigate alternative processes that could serve to avoid a reduction or lessen its impact. Staff reduction will proceed only after all reasonable alternatives have been either implemented or eliminated from consideration.
3. When circumstances necessitate staff reduction, management will determine the numbers and kinds of positions to be eliminated.

B. Guidelines Affecting Incumbent Employees
1. Nonexempt employees, excluding those in certain essential positions that may be designated by management, will be

continues

Exhibit 13-1   Model Policy and Procedure: Reduction in Force (continued)

subject to layoff generally by job assignment and by department according to staffing needs.

2. The employees working within a specific job assignment and department will be ranked using the following criteria:
   - The appropriateness of individual qualifications and experience in meeting the Hospital's needs
   - Past performance (average of the three most recent performance appraisals)
   - Disciplinary counselings or warnings within the past twelve (12) months
   - Hospital seniority.
   Each of the foregoing criteria may account for up to 25 percent of the ranking decision for an employee. From time to time, depending on circumstances and need, the Hospital may devise rating scales to facilitate employee ranking.

   After all employees within the department or job assignment are placed in rank order, selection for layoff will proceed in reverse order of the list.

3. Employees remaining in a department following a staff reduction may be subject to changes in hours, shift schedules, and work assignments as necessary.

4. Management may exercise the right to displace less senior nonexempt employees in one department with qualified nonexempt employees from another department who have greater Hospital seniority, provided this is done within similar job assignments and without significant disruption of departmental functioning.

5. Management, physicians, and other exempt positions, and certain technical and professional nonexempt positions that may be designated, are subject to position-specific reductions without regard to seniority or other factors. The principal criterion for determining the status of such positions will be their appropriateness in meeting the needs of the Hospital.

6. Any employee identified for layoff will be considered for other possibilities, such as transfer or demotion to a position in an area of need. Whenever possible the employee will be allowed to choose from available alternatives. An employee's request for reassignment to an alternative position will be honored solely at management's discretion. A displaced employee who declines an alternative position will be dismissed.

continues

**Exhibit 13-1   Model Policy and Procedure: Reduction in
Force** (continued)

Administration of Reduction

1. The department manager will identify the positions to be eliminated and furnish Administration with a list of those positions and
   the incumbent employees.
2. Administration and Human Resources will review the potentially
   affected employees proposed for possible transfer or reassignment
   to area of need, if any, and will recommend as appropriate.
3. Human Resources will submit departmental lists of employees
   recommended for layoff to the appropriate vice president and
   the president.
4. Following executive approval of layoff, Human Resources will
   coordinate with department managers to arrange for providing
   employees proper notification of termination date and information concerning terminal benefits.
5. Each affected employee will be offered an exit interview
   intended to cover:
   • Method of payout of accrued vacation time
   • Status and conversion of insurance coverage
   • Pension plan vesting, if appropriate
   • Unemployment compensation procedures
   • Reinstatement rights, if any
   • Recommendations or referrals for external placement, if any.

Other Considerations

1. Every effort will be made to eliminate the use of all temporary
   employees, whether Hospital or agency, before regular employees are considered for layoff.
2. An employee who is still in the introductory period (the first six
   months of employment) need not be ranked with others according to B.2. If such an employee's job is eliminated, the
   individual is to be considered dismissed due to lack of work.
3. A full-time employee may displace another full-time employee
   or a part-time employee, but a part-time employee may displace only another part-time employee of equal or fewer hours.
4. For employees for whom a recommendation for layoff depends
   in part on performance or disciplinary issues, there must be
   appropriate supporting documentation in the Hospital's personnel files.

Attachment: Employee Ranking Scale

continues

Exhibit 13-1   Model Policy and Procedure: Reduction in Force (continued)

Employee Ranking Scale

(a) **Qualifications/Experience**
- Still learning the job — 0
- Fully trained but limited experience — 2
- Fully trained and experienced — 4
- Cross-functional capability; fully trained in multiple areas — 6

(b) **Past Performance**
- Average of three most recent evaluations <3.5 (standard) — 0
- Average of three most recent evaluations 3.5 to 4.25 — 2
- Average of three most recent evaluations 4.26 to 4.70 — 4
- Average of three most recent evaluations >4.70 — 6

(c) **Disciplinary Counseling/Warnings** (recent 12 months)
- Multiple problems; suspended one or more times — 0
- More than two counselings, or no more than two warnings — 2
- One or two counselings, or one warning — 4
- No counselings, no warnings — 6

(d) **Seniority** (Hospital)
- Less than 1 year — 0
- 1 to 2 years — 2
- 2 to 5 years — 4
- More than 5 years — 6

NOTE: This ranking scale should be applied to groups of employees who work within the same job description engaged in the same general activities. Employees in the group should be arrayed from highest (possible 24) to lowest, with the lowest rankings receiving first consideration for reduction.

Human Resource professionals who develop reduction plans and policies are divided on whether it is best to phase reductions over a period of time or to accomplish all layoffs at once, although those favoring implementing layoffs all at once seem to have the edge. Either approach has shortcomings.

Often when layoffs are phased over a period of time, morale and productivity decrease as everyone waits for "the other shoe to drop," wondering who will go next. Teamwork becomes a far second to individual survival, and the effect spreads across the entire organization and perhaps even throughout levels of management (if the reduction is sufficiently widespread as to affect managers).

Even when the layoff is significant in numbers, there are usually far more people left working than there were workers released, and prolonged, phased reductions take their toll on the morale and attitudes of those who remain. It requires healing time for a work force to recover from a staff reduction, and the longer the reduction takes the deeper the injuries go and the longer the recovery time required. Phased layoffs are usually easier to handle administratively and easier for operating management to determine precisely what adjustments should be made, but from an employee perspective they are far more stress- and anxiety-producing than a single mass layoff.

Other Layoff Considerations

The majority of organizations employ some form *of severance policy* in conjunction with layoffs that are considered permanent; that is, reductions that do not encompass the possibility of recall to work within a reasonable period of time. Severance pay is ordinarily based on an individual's final salary in combination with length of service (e.g., one to three weeks' pay per year of service), perhaps capped at some maximum number of years. On average, health care organizations tend to offer less generous severance pay than other types of organizations.

In exchange for a severance pay arrangement—and possibly even outplacement assistance—through Human Resources, the organization may ask a departing employee to sign a *waiver of the right to sue*. In doing so the employee essentially agrees not to bring charges related to the termination in exchange for what is probably a more generous severance arrangement than would otherwise be obtainable. However, such waivers are often successfully challenged after the fact, so they are no guarantee that legal complications will be avoided.

Give all employees the *reasons for the layoff* and do so in a straightforward manner in as much detail as can be readily understood. The reasons behind most reductions in force are of course economic. It is always likely that some employees will choose not to believe the reasons they are given, but if no reasons are provided, employees will have all the more cause to feel they are being treated unfairly. Ideally employees should be kept advised of the organization's financial health on a regular basis and even reminded now and then that layoffs are possible. It is always best to avoid surprises; employees will be sufficiently shocked as it is when a layoff is announced, even if they had reason to suspect one was coming.

No Easy Time

As far as line management and Human Resources are concerned, there is nothing easy about implementing a reduction in force. However, compared with the employees who are being laid off, management and HR are far from experiencing the most difficult parts of the process.

Among employees who are laid off, feelings of anger and betrayal are normal. Terminated employees face psychological stress and economic hardship. Personal routines are disrupted, as are relationships that may have existed for years. To many individuals, the loss of a job is as traumatic as a death in the family, and surely the grieving process is parallel to that degree of loss. For all practical purposes, lives are turned inside out as individuals are thrown into a mode that some of them may never have experienced.

The overall impact of a reduction in force is eventually healed by the passage of time, especially if a measure of employment stability returns to the organization and things otherwise "settle down." Nonetheless, the initial impact is invariably stressful for both the laid-off employees and those who remain, and it may be necessary to use the employee assistance program (EAP) and other resources to help ease the transition for both laid-off staff and stressed-out survivors.

RELATED DIMENSIONS OF TERMINATION

Several other aspects of termination may involve the department manager to some extent.

Unemployment Compensation

As noted, an employee who is discharged for cause is technically not eligible for unemployment compensation, but one who is dismissed for performance-related reasons or simply laid off for lack of work or for economic reasons is considered eligible. Regardless of the reasons behind the termination, any terminated employee is free to *apply* for unemployment compensation. It costs only the time for a trip to the unemployment office to fill out a claim, and often someone the organization considered ineligible may be granted a favorable determination.

Consider an example. An individual is discharged for chronic tardiness after many counselings and warnings and following the proper application of the progressive disciplinary process. As long as policy is followed and applied consistently, the organization has every right to release the employee for not meeting the expectation of being on the job when needed. This individual is technically not eligible for unemployment compensation, but say this person applies anyway and pleads that hardship caused the inability to get to work on time—his or her supposedly regular ride has been erratic, the bus schedule keeps changing, or child care arrangements are in a state of flux. Say the unemployment office makes a determination in favor of the employee and so notifies the employer. If the employer protests the determination, there will then be a hearing, following which an administrative law judge will render a decision. Under the "hardship" circumstances just described, very often a discharged employee will be granted unemployment compensation.

Usually it is Human Resources, acting on the organization's behalf, that initially responds to any claim for unemployment compensation that arises, and HR usually makes an initial determination regarding which claims to contest and which to concede. Some Human Resources departments have taken the authoritarian stance of automatically contesting every unemployment claim, but this practice does little more than consume time and energy while generating ill will. Rather, the HR assessment of each unemployment claim should involve an honest judgment of the merits and validity of the claim, and only those claims that appear invalid or questionable should be contested.

When a claim is contested and results in a hearing before an administrative law judge, the department manager and a Human Resources representative usually attend the hearing, along with the employee and perhaps an advocate, to provide information on which a decision will eventually be based. Considering preparation and travel and waiting time, an unemployment hearing can consume several hours of a busy department manager's working life; a conscientious HR manager will be mindful of the impact on managers and will contest only those claims that honestly appear to be unwarranted.

Employee Privacy

Any termination, regardless of the reasons behind it, should be accomplished in private and in a place where the conversation is not visible to other employees (that should rule out the far corner of the cafeteria or someone's glassed-in cubicle). It is also suggested that termination be accomplished near the end of the work day so that an individual who has just been let go can leave the premises without being trapped into explanations or into answering other employees' questions about what is happening.

Any terminated employee should be afforded as much dignity as possible, although the manager may sometimes discover that doing so means walking a fine line between trust and caution. A number of distressing lessons have been learned concerning terminated employees. Some employees who have been told of their termination but were then left to their own devices to pack up and leave have caused considerable damage in a relatively short time. For example, when one organization's charitable foundation felt it necessary to lay off its full-time support person, while packing up to depart, that individual, with a few computer keystrokes, wiped out the foundation's contributor database.

Clearly some employees left to themselves will commit sabotage or vandalism out of the immediate anger generated by termination. On the other hand, some employees who were told they were terminated and were then escorted out have sued because of the humiliation experienced in the manner of departure. Juries are frequently sympathetic to the contention that defamation can result from actions as well as from words.

Sometimes Human Resources or the department manager may feel that a particular termination is sufficiently questionable to merit the presence of security personnel. If it is determined that security should be readily accessible, make the security officer's presence discreet, not especially visible but near enough for fast response if necessary.

Outplacement

If significant numbers of employees are being released in the same reduction, the organization might want to make some form of outplacement service available. Individual outplacement services are often extended as part of the severance arrangement made with a manager or a professional employee; these are individualized services intended to assist the person in preparing a resume and mounting a job search. For rank-and-file employees, group outplacement activities are often provided, and occasionally direct contacts with organizations that are known to be recruiting are supplied. Any such boost toward new employment can help lessen the feeling of betrayal or abandonment that many employees experience when laid off.

Human Resources Follow-Up

For all terminations, Human Resources representatives will address benefits issues with departing employees. This will likely include explaining the individual's continuation insurance coverage rights under the Consolidated Omnibus Budget Reconciliation Act (COBRA) and showing how application is made, explaining other insurance conversions as applicable, describing how unemployment compensation is applied for if applicable, verifying the return of property such as keys and identification badges, and perhaps securing signed releases to give out reference information. Human Resources will ordinarily also explain how remaining vacation time and applicable severance will be paid out, and whom the employee should contact with questions.

THE SURVIVORS OF A REDUCTION IN FORCE

Before, during, and immediately after a reduction in force, the people who have been subject to layoff understandably receive a great deal of attention. Often those who have been terminated receive so much attention that those who remain seem to have been forgotten. Consider that following even a 10 percent reduction in staff—a fairly large reduction by most standards—some 90 percent of employees remain. Those "survivors" must be counted on not only to keep the organization running but to also pick up the slack created by the absence of those who were let go.

It is relatively common for many among the survivors to:

- Feel overworked, if not overwhelmed, especially in the early days following the reduction, when the pinch created by the absence of some staff is most pronounced
- Experience guilt over having survived the reduction while so many others lost their jobs
- Feel distrustful of management for terminating so many of their coworkers
- Wonder how secure they are, fearing that perhaps they will be next to depart
- Experience an overall decrease in morale, productivity, and loyalty
- Feel less compelled to be at work on time or be at work at all under certain circumstances, contributing to a general increase in absenteeism and tardiness
- Consider, in a few extreme instances, and perhaps now and then carry out, acts of sabotage or violence or other disruptive behavior.

Inevitably some of the survivors of a reduction react by starting to shop around for new employment, and some critically needed staff can be lost because of the insecurity of the environment. Skilled technical and professional employees, the many "free agents" who are in demand and often feel more loyalty to their occupation than to the organization, see whatever loyalty the organization may have exhibited eroding with the reduction and are thus well positioned to be lured away by offers of "more secure" employment. A job market favorable to highly skilled professionals can cause the organization to lose some of the staff it worked so hard to protect.

The attitude among the survivors of a reduction can be particularly grim if the organization had experienced a total quality management (TQM) program or other motivational program during recent years. These programs, launched and pursued with much promotional activity and a strong emphasis on the value of employee participation, deliver a message loud and clear to each employee: You are important; you and your contributions are essential to our continued success; you are needed. Then, not long after hearing how much they are needed, along comes a downturn in the organization's fortunes and a necessary reduction in force that delivers the contrary message: But we no longer need nearly as many of you as before. Often when a significant reduction in force follows a TQM implementation, the effect is more demoralizing than if the employees had never heard of total quality management.

Following a significant layoff, it is important for top management to be openly supportive of those who remain and to be visibly active in the effort to help the survivors adjust to the changes and return to normal operations. It will of course be helpful if employees can be given reasonable assurance that no more layoffs are anticipated. Because this is what so many of the survivors want to hear, it may be all too easy to simply tell them so, but this is a message that should be delivered only if it can be done with nearly complete confidence. One can imagine the reactions if employees are assured that there will be no more layoffs, only to experience another reduction within a few months.

Management at all levels, as well as Human Resources, can provide valuable support to the survivors of a reduction in force by stressing training and education as people attempt to settle in to new or altered roles. Specifically, this can be an appropriate time to consider an emphasis on training in managing time in one's new role, managing stress, and coping with change. Anything that can be done to smooth the return to a sense of "business as usual," to allay the fears of the work force and turn their primary interest from survival and security back toward service to patients, will be helpful.

During the recovery period following a reduction in force, it is important for the department manager to remain in close communication with the group. This can be a tough time for the manager; employees will have questions, many of which will be unanswerable. Employees will perhaps be stressed out, worried, and demoralized. As "just another employee," the department manager is subject to all of these same negative influences. Yet if the manager is to have any chance at all of keeping the department's employees upbeat and willing to produce despite of what is occurring around them, the manager must set the example by remaining upbeat in the face of potential discouragement. This is no easy task, but it may help to remember that quite likely the outlook of an entire group of people—the department's employees—often hinges on the outlook of a single person—the manager.

Discussion Points

1. Explain fully the defining differences between the modes of termination referred to as *dismissal* and *discharge*.
2. Discuss the timing of a general layoff in terms of whether you believe it is better to implement a sizeable reduction in a single action or to phase it in over a period of weeks or months. Provide reasons for your recommendations.
3. Using a hypothetical department in a health care organization—the kind of service rendered is up to you (nursing, food service, radiology, etc.)—identify the steps you would recommend taking *before* laying off employees.
4. Describe the principal advantages and disadvantages of implementing a voluntary early retirement program.
5. Describe the concept of *constructive discharge* and provide an example.
6. Explain why some form of seniority is the most frequently applied criterion in identifying employees for layoff.
7. Discuss why it is necessary to pay particular attention to the employees who are retained following a reduction in force.

These survivors still have their jobs; what do they have to be concerned with?

8. Consider whether employees who are laid off should be expected to leave on the day they are notified or should be allowed to work out a reasonable period of notice. Provide reasons for your choice.

9. Describe specifically why mergers and other affiliations often lead to the consolidation of positions and reduction of the work force.

10. Discuss whether a manager should be able to use the reason of a reduction in force to rid the department of its less effective employees. Why, or why not?

11. If employee performance and behavior are used as partial criteria for determining who is subject to layoff (as in the Model Policy and Procedure presented in Exhibit 13-1), describe what will have to be in place to minimize the possibility of such terminations being overturned by legal action. Why?

12. Once a reduction plan has been completed to the extent of identifying all employees marked for layoff, explain what must be done—usually through Human Resources—before the plan is implemented. Why?

13. Assume that a significant number of employees of a particular skill—registered nurses, laboratory technologists, etc.— are designated for layoff as part of a major reduction in services. Identify as many ways as possible that the organization can assist these workers following termination.

14. Explain why it is advisable (perhaps necessary) to provide a one-on-one meeting in Human Resources for each employee terminated in a workforce reduction.

15. Discuss whether it is ever advisable to allow an employee who is about to be discharged for cause to resign "for the record." Why, or why not?

NOTES

[1]Chris Serb, "Is Remaking the Hospital Making Money?" *Hospitals and Health Networks,* Vol. 72, No. 14, July 20, 1998, p. 32.

[2]Ibid., p. 33.

CHAPTER 14

See You in Court:
Involvement in Legal Action

This chapter—

- Comments on the apparently increasing tendency of employees and ex-employees to seek recourse in legal processes
- Reviews the legal basis for the majority of actions brought by employees and former employees
- Establishes the potential for involvement in a legal action as an inherent aspect of the department manager's role
- Identifies the strongest deterrent to legal complaints as a sound, humane employee relations philosophy
- Indicates the initial steps to be taken when the organization receives a legal complaint
- Reviews the process for dealing with a legal complaint
- Outlines the involvement of Human Resources and the department manager in the legal process of *discovery*
- Provides specific guidelines for providing deposition testimony
- Provides guidelines for the department manager in coexisting in the department with an employee-plaintiff while a complaint is pending resolution.

ANYONE CAN FILE, ANYONE CAN SUE

Top management is usually concerned, and rightly so, with the likelihood of legal entanglements, not only because of the costs and time involved but also because of the attendant stress and aggravation. The chief executive officer (CEO) of a sizable health care organization, especially a hospital, has every reason to be concerned with legal actions; Human Resources may experience legal actions involving employment, and the department manager may occasionally be involved in one, but the CEO sees them all—the occasional employment actions, and the far more frequent actions involving charges of medical malpractice.

One particular hospital CEO used to demand of his key staff, specifically his director of Human Resources, "I want this problem taken care of in such a way that nobody can sue us." Although it is possible to "take care of" many matters in such a way that nobody would be likely to sue *and win*, this particular CEO never completely understood that there is no way to guarantee that no one will sue.

Unfortunately, it cannot even be guaranteed, even under the most favorable of conditions, that if a particular party sues, he or she absolutely cannot win. Time and again cases that have appeared to be guaranteed winners for the organization have been known to go the other way in the hands of judge or jury.

Essentially anyone can sue, or can file a charge in another venue (such as an advocacy agency), and the organization is obliged to become involved. Any employee who can visit the state's human rights division or the Equal Employment Opportunity Commission (EEOC), tell a reasonable story, and fill out (with help) a written complaint can begin an action against an employer. Any employee who can get an attorney sufficiently interested to take on a particular issue can file a lawsuit. When either occurs, the organization has no choice: Any legal complaint received must be answered.

This chapter addresses the involvement of the department manager in legal actions, primarily administrative complaints and lawsuits brought by present or former employees. The involvement of Human Resources, Administration, and legal counsel will be addressed for the sake of understanding the overall process, but the focus will be on the department manager's involvement.

THE LEGAL ENVIRONMENT

Legal action is more and more becoming the recourse of aggrieved employees. The causes of this increasing employee interest and involvement in legal action appear to be:

- Proliferation of laws affecting all aspects of employment
- Growing awareness of individuals' rights

- Unrest and uncertainty in health care
- Increasing publicity concerning legal complaints, including news of increasingly larger monetary awards.

The key laws (see Chapter 3 for more details) that give rise to legal complaints brought by employees and former employees are:

- *Title VII of the Civil Rights Act of 1964.* A large number of employment-related legal actions involve charges of unlawful discrimination of various kinds, usually claiming violation of some aspect of Title VII of the Civil Rights Act of 1964. Since this legislation established the EEOC as an enforcement agency and was also responsible for the establishment of state divisions of human rights, Title VII essentially drives all administrative complaints alleging discrimination and the majority of employment-related lawsuits.

  One of the most active areas involving charges against employers, and certainly one of the most publicized, is sexual harassment. Sexual harassment is legally considered a form of sex discrimination, so such charges ordinarily fall under Title VII.
- *Age Discrimination in Employment Act.* Numerous charges of age discrimination in hiring, job retention, compensation, and all other terms, conditions, and privileges of employment are filed citing the ADEA, presently also enforced by the EEOC. In terms of frequency of charges and visibility through publicity, age discrimination remains second only to sexual harassment.
- *Pregnancy Discrimination Act.* Although claims are not filed citing this legislation, this law was responsible for defining pregnancy discrimination as a form of sex discrimination and bringing it under Title VII.
- *Americans With Disabilities Act.* Some charges of discrimination on the basis of disability are filed under Title VII and some are filed under ADA; in some actions both laws are mentioned. On some occasions a job applicant will be attempting to secure a "reasonable accommodation," perhaps with the definition of what is "reasonable" in dispute. Sometimes an applicant will claim the ability to perform the major functions of a job, charging that the job was denied because an impairment prevents performance of a minor or non-essential activity.

- *Civil Rights Act of 1991.* This act put more force behind some dimensions of the Civil Rights Act of 1964, provided for jury trials in certain instances where they were not previously used, and increased potential damage awards. This had the effect of increasing the likelihood of longer and costlier legal processes and costlier penalties.
- *Family and Medical Leave Act.* The disagreements and occasional charges arising from application of this law often involve an employee's claim of (1) having been denied leave to which he or she is entitled, or (2) returning from leave and finding that the position "held" was neither the original position nor a fully "equivalent" position.

Any manager in the organization can be drawn into a legal action, and the manager will have no choice about participating. Participation, especially in a lawsuit that runs its complete course including trial, can be stressful and time-consuming.

PREVENTING COMPLAINTS

It is not possible to provide a list of steps a manager can take to guarantee that he or she will never receive a legal complaint. Nonetheless, preventive maintenance consists of what the manager should have been doing all along: treating all employees equally and with respect and regard for each as an individual and as a whole person. The best prevention for employment-related legal complaints is a sound, humane employee relations approach.

Approaches that can help prevent complaints or that can be useful in properly and thoroughly addressing those complaints that do arise include:

- A progressive disciplinary process that is fair and consistent in its applications to all employees and for which all documentation is timely and complete
- Thorough documentation of all efforts to work positively with substandard performers
- Examination with Human Resources of the legal implications of all proposed personnel actions
- All forms generated concerning employees and all other pertinent documentation completed, signed, and filed as required, with extraneous copies or obsolete versions properly discarded

- Objective and consistently maintained anecdotal note files that are regularly purged of duplicative or nonessential information.

Legal actions often require the production of large amounts of paper. As noted in Chapter 12, Employee Documentation: Shoulds and Should-Nots for the Manager, documents that are incomplete, unsigned, undated, unreadable, or just plain missing simply add to the manager's burden.

WHEN A COMPLAINT ARRIVES

A legal complaint involving either a past or present employee (or multiple individuals) will arise in one of two ways.

The employee may file with the EEOC or the state division of human rights. Filing costs the employee nothing, and even a relatively thin complaint is likely to be accepted by the agency. Once the complaint is accepted and delivered, the organization (usually through Human Resources but sometimes with considerable involvement of the department manager) is obligated to expend time and effort preparing an answer and subsequently participating in some aspect of the agency's investigation of the complaint.

The other route through which a complaint may arise is the filing of a lawsuit. Anyone who can interest an attorney in his or her story is free to sue. Doing so may cost the individual something up front; a considerable percentage of attorneys do not ordinarily offer contingency-fee arrangements in employment-related actions.

The majority of employment-related actions begin with a filing with EEOC or Human Rights. This less formal route is less costly for all concerned and often considerably faster (but can still drag on for months or even years). When an individual files with the EEOC, that agency ordinarily refers the complaint to the state human rights agency for initial processing. Thus, the usual route for an administrative complaint (as opposed to a lawsuit) to enter is via Human Rights.

In some organizations it is a firm policy to involve an attorney as soon as an administrative complaint arrives. In others, if the initial investigation of the complaint involves the agency only, the organization will choose to use internal resources such as Human Resources, Risk Management, or Administration to coordinate the organization's response and relate to the agency without using an attorney. However, if the employee filing the agency complaint also engages an attorney to see the complaint through, the organization had best use an attorney from the start. An employee's use of an attorney to drive an administrative complaint usually indicates an advanced level of seriousness, so it is best to react seriously. Also, it is probably not the best choice to put an administrative complaint in the hands of in-house legal counsel if the house attorney is a legal generalist; Human Rights and EEOC complaints, as well as employment-related lawsuits, are best served by an attorney who specializes in employment law.

In some states the aggrieved employee must initially choose between filing an administrative complaint or filing a lawsuit in state court. When the employee chooses one of these routes, the choice generally closes the other route.

An individual must file an administrative complaint with EEOC before beginning a federal lawsuit. Once a complaint has been with EEOC for six months and no action has been taken (not at all uncommon), the employee can request (usually through an attorney) and receive notification of the right to sue in federal court.

A particular charge should be considered neither more nor less serious by virtue of being filed in federal court, state court, or with an administrative agency. Even Human Rights may have the power to order back pay or reinstatement to a job or the payment of monetary damages upon a ruling favorable to the complainant. The organization's response to EEOC or Human Rights must be thorough and accurate; anything at all involved in addressing the charge at administrative level may surface later in federal court.

It is not necessarily in the organization's best interests to fight every complaint all the way. It rarely pays to automatically dig in and resist; it is necessary to closely examine all elements of the complaint and all implications of the charges before deciding upon the most appropriate course of action. There are always at least three choices: (1) concede to the complaint and grant what is demanded, (2) negotiate a mutually acceptable solution, or (3) dig in and fight.

THE PROCESS

The department manager should have a basic understanding of the process the organization will follow once a complaint has been received.

The Internal Coordinator

One individual within the organization should be charged with the responsibility for coordinating all involvement in resolving a legal complaint. Depending on whether the organization is dealing with an administrative complaint or a lawsuit, this responsibility could involve a great deal of necessary activity. The coordinator will be involved in making certain that the appropriate people—invariably including the department manager—are lined up for depositions and perhaps court appearances. There are often many issues of timing, as the schedules of all others involved are ordinarily subject to the schedules of attorneys and, later, the court calendar. Frequently a substantial amount of document retrieval and copying is necessary.

Depending largely on the size and structure of the organization, the case coordinator may be in-house legal counsel, the risk manager, a Human Resources professional, a line manager, or a member of Administration (assistant or associate administrator, perhaps). In addition to arranging schedules and securing documents, the coordinator works with the primary attorney to ensure continuity throughout the case, keep top management advised of status and progress, and convey management's questions and concerns to the attorney.

As top management's frustration mounts, especially in a lengthy (which also means costly) case, some tendency to "shoot the messenger" may arise; thus, the coordinator must be diplomatic as well as thorough. In relating to top management, the coordinator should be aware at all times that management needs information as it accrues, even detail by detail. What management decidedly does not need are long periods of silence followed by surprises. Top management does not like surprises, especially costly ones.

The Internal Investigation

The organization's initial response to a complaint should be to conduct an internal investigation to clarify the issues involved in the complaint and to develop a sense of its validity. In addition to the internal coordinator, the investigation will involve Human Resources, possibly Administration, and probably the department manager and a number of other employees. The investigation will include interviews with all named or involved parties except the complainant, who must now be dealt with through his or her representative, whether administrative agency or attorney. All pertinent documents will also be reviewed.

The internal investigation is a time for absolute, perhaps even brutal, honesty; it is *not* a time to simply assume the organization is in the right and to charge on with a defense. It is necessary to look for errors or instances of wrongdoing or incorrect judgment on the organization's part, to avoid attempting to rationalize mistakes or cover them up.

This is the time to bring all real problems out in the open for all concerned within the organization. Brutal honesty at this stage may help establish an appropriate case strategy and may save time, legal costs, and aggravation. If it indeed appears that the organization has committed an infraction or that one of its agents has acted in a discriminatory manner, the best course of action may be to attempt to negotiate a resolution before the legal bills begin to mount.

Although management may elect to pursue the internal investigation without yet involving legal counsel, there can be times when early involvement of the organization's labor counsel may be appropriate. A case that is complicated or in which emotional involvement is high on one or both sides could be on the road to becoming a lawsuit. Throughout the internal investigation it is necessary to remember that in the event a lawsuit is filed, any documentation generated during the investigation—interview transcripts, notes, whatever—can be demanded through the discovery process unless protected by legal privilege. If an attorney is directing the investigation, chances are that the resulting documentation can be protected by attorney-client privilege.

Settlement Decisions

During the pursuit of a complaint, settlement offers may be made or requested. Details of settlement offers usually come through the organization's attorney to the case coordinator, who will then review them with top management. The attorney may make a recommendation concerning settlement, but a decision to settle and on what terms belongs to management. Chances are that the department manager will have no voice in accepting or rejecting a settlement decision.

Probably one of the most difficult aspects of a legal action for persons who are not ordinarily involved in such matters is to seriously consider settlement when they are absolutely convinced they have done no wrong. There is perhaps a natural tendency to feel that paying any amount in the way of settlement is an admission of wrongdoing. However, it makes little sense to vow, as so many who have felt wrongly charged have done, that they will never be made to pay anything.

If a charge can be shown to be frivolous early in the process, perhaps it will be thrown out of the legal system. If it is retained, however, it must either be pursued for the entire distance—or settled.

Settlement is a practical decision. As unfair as doing so may seem, paying what could be simply a token amount to get rid of the charge can be far more economical than going through a trial. When "winning" means time, frustration, and significant legal fees, settlement (if reasonable) can be the wisest course of action.

In deciding on settlement, it helps to have developed a strong feeling about where the case appears to be heading. Even if it seems clear that the organization is without fault, there must be legal proof. Also keep in mind that if the case goes to trial, juries often tend to side with the employee regardless of the strength of the evidence. Given a choice, plaintiffs' attorneys invariably prefer jury trials because of the tendency of juries to see the contest as small versus large, that is, the individual versus a corporate entity.

Regarding settlement, it is also necessary to consider the possible effects of publicity, both within and outside of the organization. Internally, the organization may be cautious about an early settlement that appears to give a complainant a victory because other employees may be encouraged to sue. Externally, there are issues of the organization's image to consider.

The best times to settle are usually:

- Early, before either the plaintiff or the organization has invested much time, money, and energy in pursuing the case, and when perhaps the plaintiff will go away for a modest payment.
- Immediately following discovery, when both sides have seen the evidence and each may have a much clearer indication of the direction the case could be taking.
- After a motion for summary judgment has been disposed of but before actually beginning trial. If portions of the case have been dismissed, the relative merits of the remaining charges may be clearer, so the parties may be more amenable to a settlement.

Discovery

Discovery is that period in the conduct of a lawsuit during which depositions of various parties are taken and documents are called forth and examined. It is at the beginning of discovery that the organization will likely be in receipt of the *notice to produce* (as described in Chapter 12, Employee Documentation: Shoulds and Should-Nots for the Manager).

Discovery could conceivably surface any document ever created concerning the complaining employee or in any way related to the charge. The manager is again reminded to complete each and every document that is ever filed in such a way that the writer or the organization would not be embarrassed should it become public.

Business must go on as usual while a case is underway. If the case involves an employee who is still within the organization, each piece of new documentation created concerning that person should be reviewed with legal counsel. This is a particularly sensitive time for the department manager. On the one hand, the manager must continue to treat all employees in the department equally and hold them to the same standards of behavior; on the other hand, the manager should be aware that any perception on the part of the complaining employee of being "picked on" could result in further charges, specifically charges of retaliation for having filed a complaint.

While a case is in progress, any documentation prepared specifically at the request of the organization's attorney should be identified as such. This kind of material can often be protected from discovery by attorney-client privilege.

Once a complaint has been received, whether an administrative complaint or a lawsuit, no documents that are in any way related to the case should be destroyed. If documents are destroyed after the notice to produce is received, the organization may be liable for legal sanctions. Also, even if documentation that has been disposed of was absolutely harmless, the mere fact of its destruction can create the perception of a cover-up. All too often when documentation is missing, the worst is assumed.

For an administrative complaint, the term "discovery" is not generally applied. Rather, when an administrative complaint is received, it will include an information request, which the employer is expected to fulfill. The information requested will vary with the kind of complaint and the individuals involved, but as a rule it can be expected to include pertinent personnel files, job applications, job descriptions, other documents as specified, and a narrative response to the specific charges in the complaint itself

In pursuing an administrative complaint, investigators from the agency will interview various persons at the workplace or will call them to the agency's office for interviews. In this manner, the agency's investigators will gather information for a recommendation. If the complaint is a lawsuit, the more formal, time-consuming route of depositions will be followed. Although depositions are usually taken in attorneys' offices, they are done with the deposed parties under oath and with full transcripts generated exactly as if it were testimony given in a courtroom. Present for depositions are, at a minimum, the attorneys representing both sides, a court reporter (who also has the power to swear in witnesses), and the individual being deposed; also present may be a representative of the organization (usually the case coordinator) and perhaps the plaintiff(s).

Any employees called to testify, as well as any expert witnesses engaged by the defense, will be prepared for deposition testimony by the organization's attorney. It is at this point that the department manager is likely to become involved. A great many discrimination charges involve allegations of how an individual has been dealt with relative to some aspect of employment, so the individual's manager is almost always called upon (if not also named individually in the charge, which is relatively common). Therefore, the department manager is likely to be deposed.

The individual being deposed should:

- Listen carefully to each question before responding. If a question seems unclear, ask for clarification before answering.
- Do not volunteer extraneous information. Answer each question exactly as it is asked, with no expansion or embellishment.
- If what is asked seems to include more than a single question, ask to have the questions separated and restated.
- Do not guess at answers. Often the most honest and accurate answer is "I don't know" or "I don't recall."
- Take time to think about the question and deliver a thoughtful response. Do not allow yourself to be rushed.
- Take care to avoid being trapped into admissions of wrongdoing in response to accusations that are framed as questions. (Your organization's attorney will help guard against this.)
- Do not be flippant or sarcastic, and do not under any circumstances try to be funny.

Deposition requires people to be away from their jobs for a few hours to several days, with as much or even more time having to be spent preparing to be deposed.

Discovery can lead to more discovery as the case progresses. For instance, say there has already been a notice to produce, and considerable documentation has been provided. Depositions occur, and during a deposition the plaintiff's attorney learns of some possibly relevant documentation that had not originally been requested. There follows another document request, more copies, and subsequently more deposition questioning. This sometimes goes on to the extent of a plaintiff's attorney conducting what might be described as a "fishing expedition," continuing to dig more deeply in the apparent hope of finding something incriminating. On occasion such "expeditions" have to be curtailed by judicial order.

Conclusions and Non-Conclusions

When the administrative agency has completed its investigation, it issues a determination. The determination and the reasons for it are then communicated in writing to both the complainant and the organization. The determination will take one of two forms: *probable cause* or *no probable cause*.

A probable cause determination means that the agency has decided there is enough evidence to indicate probable cause that discrimination has occurred; in other words, that it is likely or at least possible that discrimination has occurred and thus there is some substance to the charges. This determination may be followed by a suggested solution, or the agency may proceed directly into a formal legal action and sue the employer on behalf of the complainant. The organization may of course appeal the probable cause determination to the state human rights authority.

A determination of no probable cause means just that: The agency has decided there is no probable cause to believe that discrimination has occurred. Following this determination, the complainant has a specific amount of time in which to appeal the determination. As with an employer's appeal of a probable cause ruling, a complainant's appeal is heard at the state level, bypassing the regional human rights office that made the determination. When a complainant decides to proceed with an appeal, it is usually with the assistance of an attorney.

A lawsuit that is not resolved by settlement along the way will eventually go to court as a civil (as opposed to criminal) action. Depending on the nature of the complaint and the law or laws under which it is filed, the case may be heard by a judge alone or by a jury. Plaintiffs often have a choice, but plaintiffs' attorneys almost always request a jury trial. As noted, in cases involving employment matters, civil court juries tend to be more sympathetic toward plaintiffs. Even plaintiffs who have not come across as complete innocents are often awarded some nominal amount because of the perceived "David and Goliath" character of the conflict and the general belief that a corporation can afford it.

Although a final-sounding verdict may be rendered at the end of a trial, the matter is usually far from over. There are legal motions to follow (e.g., motion to vacate the verdict) that must be heard and addressed, and there are the very nearly inevitable appeals. It can be months, and often years, after the rendering of a verdict before any award is actually paid and the entire matter can be considered closed.

LIVING WITH AN ACTIVE CASE

As noted earlier, when the employee who has filed the charge remains working in the organization, the department manager has to be especially careful to avoid any appearance of differential treatment. Charges can be added to the complaint along the way; it is not unusual for the employee to claim that some adverse action was taken in retaliation for having filed a complaint. Usually both the manager and the employee become more sensitive to the actions of the other, making it difficult for the manager, for example, to deliver a warning for some instance of behavior or even to deliver some deserved criticism.

In addition to having any personnel action involving the complaining employee checked out with legal counsel before implementation, most significant personnel actions involving anyone in the department should likewise be examined. This especially applies if promotions or other enhancements of pay or status are underway; there may be no direct action affecting the complaining employee, but that person may then claim to have been bypassed because of having filed a complaint. All in all, the manager and the complaining employee will be working under a somewhat strained relationship.

To keep the likelihood of retaliation charges to a practical minimum, only those who have a genuine need to know should be made aware of the complaint and the status of the case. When people ask about the case, as they are bound to when they read of it in the newspaper, it is best for the manager to respond by stating that active litigation cannot be discussed. The department manager, whether named as a defendant or not, should not speak about the case with anyone except the organization's attorney, the case coordinator, and top management as necessary. In many instances there will be a legal order forbidding the manager to talk about the case except with those who have a vested interest in the process. However, no one can restrain the plaintiff from talking about the case should he or she wish to do so.

As the case goes on, those who are involved will attempt to conduct business as usual. This is often no problem; there are usually long periods of time during which nothing is happening. But then there are highly disruptive, and completely unavoidable, periods of concentrated demands.

Relationships can change in the department over the course of a lengthy case. Tension and stress can take their toll on the manager, and if the manager's resentment is visible the tension can be communicated to the remainder of the staff. The complaining employee may sometimes behave as though wielding a measure of power over the manager, knowing that he or she need only make a simple telephone call to place the manager in danger of a retaliation charge.

Other employees throughout the organization are usually watching the progress of the case, some of them waiting for some simple sign of encouragement that they can interpret as an invitation to submit their own complaints.

The department manager is advised not to try to maintain a record of his or her own involvement in the case. It may be difficult if not impossible to keep personal opinion out of such a record, and its very existence would simply provide the plaintiff's attorney with one more record to be demanded. It is likely that the case coordinator will maintain a complete chronological record of the entire case.

Nearly all legal complaints seem to take longer to resolve than we feel they ought to. Even a seemingly simple administrative complaint can drag on for months. The employee advocacy agencies invariably have significant backlogs of work facing them, and as far as the courts are concerned, it is not unusual to see a backlog of several years' worth of cases awaiting their time in court. The greater the lapse of time between the charge and the trial, the more difficult the process becomes—some people who might be required as witnesses have trouble enough recalling what was said and done last week, let alone five or six years ago. Yet the process will continue to hinge upon the availability of the courts and the schedules of the attorneys.

Discussion Points

1. Consider whether there is any truth in the contention that "anyone can sue." Why is this so?
2. Describe the precautions you believe would be necessary for a manager who must continue working day-to-day with an employee who is in the process of suing the organization.
3. Write a paragraph describing why you believe today's employees are more inclined to take legal action against their employers than were their counterparts of years past.
4. Explain in detail what is meant by the claim that many cases, perhaps an overwhelming majority, are won or lost by the organization well before a complaint is ever filed.
5. Describe the fundamental differences between a *lawsuit* and an *administrative complaint*, and describe how the latter can become the former.
6. Discuss when it is advisable to pursue an administrative complaint internally without benefit of legal counsel, and when legal counsel should be involved from the start.
7. Explain why the internal investigation of a complaint is considered "a time for absolute, perhaps even brutal, honesty." What should be done if this process suggests wrongdoing by the organization?
8. Explain why one of the best times to consider settlement is following completion of all "discovery" but before the actual trial begins.
9. Identify the hazards inherent in "cleaning out old documentation" or "shaping up the files" after a *notice to produce* has been received.
10. When you are called upon to give testimony via deposition, consider whether it is in your organization's best interests for you to elaborate on your every answer to the extent of as much factual detail as you can provide. Why, or why not?
11. Define what is meant by a determination of *probable cause* following investigation of an administrative complaint, and specify what is likely to follow such a determination.
12. Thoroughly explain why it is often to the organization's disadvantage to go to trial before a jury.

PART V
Other Human Resources Concerns

CHAPTER 15

Avoiding—or Dealing with—a Union

This chapter—

- Briefly surveys the history of unionization in general and in health care in particular
- Offers a number of reasons why employees turn to unions, especially in health care today
- Reviews the reasons why organizational management ordinarily prefers to remain union-free
- Reviews health care's unique treatment under prevailing labor law
- Identifies the various bargaining units possible in an organized health care facility
- Describes the department manager's role in the union organizing process
- Reviews the visible signs of union organizing
- Describes the activity occurring following the arrival of a petition for a representation election
- Reviews what managers can or cannot legally say or do during a union organizing drive
- Provides advice to the department manager in dealing with a union day-to-day
- Describes the process by which employees can attempt to decertify an existing bargaining unit.

UNIONS: HEALTH CARE AND ELSEWHERE

For years, many who worked in health care behaved as though the health care industry was recession-proof and essentially layoff-proof. As we learned in the closing decades of the twentieth century, nothing could be farther from the truth. Financial pressures, mergers and other affiliations, and the proliferation of health care systems have changed health care from an arena in which employment could be considered relatively secure to one in which job security is fully as elusive as it is in many other businesses. When faced with insecurity and uncertainty in an environment they had traditionally regarded as stable, some employees will turn toward labor unions.

For a number of years union membership has been steadily declining in the aggregate work force of the United States; at the same time union membership in the health care industry has been increasing. In 1945, American union membership reached its peak, accounting for some 36 percent of the work force. Late in the year 2000, union membership totaled about 13.9 percent of the work force, the lowest level of union membership in the country since the National Labor Relations Act was passed in 1935. It is estimated that organized labor must add 250,000 to 500,000 new members per year just to keep pace with the annual attrition in manufacturing jobs.[1] As a consequence of such continuing losses and the perceived need to compensate for them, unions are listening carefully to health care workers and high-tech workers.

Especially susceptible to organizing pressure are direct caregivers, particularly nurses. Dissatisfaction with pay and increasingly stressful work conditions, aggravated by a shortage of nurses at hospitals across the country, are spurring job actions and the formation of nurses' unions. In 2000, 19 percent of the country's 1.3 million hospital nurses were unionized, up from 17 percent in 1999 and 16 percent in 1990.[2]

The Department of Health and Human Services predicts a shortage of 400,000 nurses by the year 2020. Although the number of registered nurses has increased by 39 percent since the last half of the 1990s, an increasing number are choosing not to work in hospitals or nursing homes. Rather, some two of every five new nurses are opting for easier, better-paying jobs with health maintenance organizations or pharmaceutical companies.[3] And the financial pressures holding down salaries and staffing in hospitals are likely to continue for some time; according to the American Hospital Association, fully a third of all hospitals operate at a loss.

Why Workers Go Union

When unions are organizing or when they are striking or threatening to strike, we hear a great deal about the monetary demands being made of employers. Certainly economic issues always figure prominently in a union's demands of employers and promises to employees, but it is primarily insecurity that encourages workers to turn to unions in the first place. Mounting health care layoffs from mergers, acquisitions, and fiscal belt-tightening have been causing many workers to look toward unions as their job security is shaken.

Management behavior, and especially some of management's mistakes and erroneous assumptions, can drive employees toward unions. For example, in assuming that employees' primary concerns are economic, management often blinds itself to the real reasons for employee dissatisfaction. Top management often seems to believe that most of what troubles employees could be fixed by giving them more money. Frequently, however, economic reasons lag far behind other reasons in causing employees to seek union representation. Insecurity and lack of communication are significant drivers of employee unrest. At all times employees want someone to listen to them, and this desire is strongest when conditions are unsettled and they are feeling threatened. If they perceive that no one in the organization is willing to listen to them, they will turn toward whomever demonstrates a willingness to listen and promises to help them. Union organizers are all too willing to be the ones who listen.

Another of top management's classic errors is to assume that because they hear little or nothing to the contrary, everything is fine among the ranks of employees. Information, especially valid, pertinent information, does not readily travel upward in the organizational structure. There are numerous organizational obstacles to the upward flow of information, and if relationships are weakened by distrust and uncertainty, little of relevance will find its way to the top. In a great many organizations (perhaps the majority), top management has very little idea what is on the minds of the people at the bottom of the structure.

Another mistake that top management frequently commits is to assume that all first-line supervisors and middle managers are automatically, by virtue of their positions, on the side of management when a union beckons. A great many lower-level managers are themselves one step up from the ranks, and many have never been made to feel like they are true managers and may in fact never have been treated as such by higher management. Often it is not until a union comes calling that higher management learns the price of not having treated its supervisors and middle managers as full-fledged members of management.

Top management also often makes a grave mistake by shutting the lower levels of management out entirely when union organizing occurs. Top management may understandably be sensitive to the possibility of supervisors inadvertently committing unfair labor practices or making other legal mistakes, so the initial tendency may be to keep the supervisors out of the process while organizing is occurring. However, the first-line supervisors, who manage the people who do the hands-on work, are in a position to be the strongest, most direct communication links between the workers and higher management. So much of a union organizing campaign, for both union and management, is communication; in insulating and isolating the first-line supervisors, management may be stifling its best communication channels.

Surely workers will sometimes go in the direction of a union because of economic concerns, and we can be certain that no matter what brought the union in, once it is in place and negotiations begin, there will be economic items on the table. But if all other factors are satisfactory, economics alone will drive union interest only if the economic disparity is dramatic. Otherwise, employees may turn toward a union if:

- For whatever reason (e.g., merger, reengineering, active layoffs), people are made to feel insecure about their employment and uncertain about future prospects.
- Major changes in organizational structure, management, operating requirements, job content, and equipment are made without notice or explanation.
- Significant changes in upper management alter the prevailing style of management from an open or consultative approach to authoritarian or autocratic management.
- Employees are given little or no information about the organization's financial status or its plans or intentions, and key decisions affecting employees' jobs and careers are made in isolation from employees' true needs.
- Instances of employee dissatisfaction are ignored or overlooked.

- Employees rarely receive feedback from management in response to their questions, complaints, and concerns, and the little feedback they do receive is negative.

Why Management Wants to Remain Non-Union

Management generally wants the organization to remain non-union for a variety of reasons, primarily to maintain greater latitude in running the operation and managing employees. When a union is in place, the terms of a contract must be followed; by dictating how certain things must be done, these terms ordinarily place limitations on certain management processes.

Unions increase the costs of doing business and thus increase the costs that must ultimately be borne by consumers. Increases in wages and benefits gained through negotiations are far from the only increases attributable to a union. For example, the costs of paying the organization's labor counsel and maintaining a labor relations function can mount up considerably. From management's point of view, the union adds cost and effort to running the health care organization without providing any enhancement of patient care.

A union can drastically realign communication relationships within the organization. Without a union, communication (at least theoretically) can flow directly between management and employees. With a union in place, some of that information must now flow through the union. This has the effect of interjecting a third party into what would otherwise be a two-party relationship, and in the case of a union it is a third party that has an agenda of its own.

Once in place, a union has as a major objective in *staying* in place. The union can stay in place over the long run (and continue to collect its dues and assessments) only by reasonably establishing its value to the employees. One way in which a union establishes its supposed value is by encouraging a level of distrust between employees and management; if relations between employees and management are completely open and cordial and satisfactory in all respects, the union wouldn't be needed. From management's point of view, therefore, the union is an extraneous element that causes extra expense and aggravation and makes operations more difficult by virtue of being a self-perpetuating entity with its own agenda.

Too often a management group has been late in learning the value of positive labor relations. It is sometimes only after a union has appeared on the scene that management begins to grasp some simple truths: If employees are treated fairly, communicated with openly and honestly, and provided with salary and benefits comparable to those provided by the local competition, chances are they will never turn to a union.

THE LEGAL FRAMEWORK AND HEALTH CARE'S UNIQUE TREATMENT

The National Labor Relations Act (NLRA) of 1935, commonly known as the Wagner Act, is the basis of most of the labor law in the United States. This act guarantees the right of employees to join unions and engage in collective bargaining, as well as the right to refuse to do so. The NLRA was amended in 1947 by the Taft-Hartley Act.

Originally the Wagner Act put clout in the hands of the unions, and it stopped many of the harsh practices of employers that formerly prevailed. After a few years, however, it began to appear that too much clout rested with the unions, so steps were taken to try to achieve a better balance between labor and management. The Taft-Hartley Act was essentially an attempt to level the playing field by returning some clout to employers and at the same time making unions more accountable.

The NLRA (i.e., the Wagner Act as amended by the Taft-Hartley Act) is enforced by the National Labor Relations Board (NLRB), a governmental agency created specifically for that purpose.

From passage of Taft-Hartley in 1947 up until 1975, not-for-profit health care institutions were exempt from all provisions of federal labor law. During that period, only the labor laws of the various states applied to such organizations. However, in 1975 the Taft-Hartley Act was amended to include not-for-profit health care organizations as covered employers. The 1975 amendments:

- Defined health care institutions fairly broadly to include any hospital, convalescent hospital, health maintenance organization (HMO), clinic, nursing home, extended care facility, or any other institution devoted to the sick, infirm, or aged
- Established the legal notification period for intended negotiations of renewals or modifications of contracts of 90 days (in all other industries this period is 60 days)

- Stated that the Federal Mediation and Conciliation Service had to be notified 60 days before the expiration of a contract (in all other industries the requirement is for 30 days' advance notification)
- Stated that the union could be required to participate in the mediation process as necessary for both initial contracts and contract renewals (no such requirement pertains to other industries)
- Requires that the union provide a 10-day advance notification of a strike, picketing, or any other concerted refusal to work (again, no such requirement pertains to unions in other industries)
- Stated that if there is a work stoppage or the threat of a work stoppage that could be disruptive of patient care delivery, the Federal Mediation and Conciliation Service can order an impartial board of inquiry to investigate the dispute and report its findings (no such provision for other industries)
- Stated that health care employees belonging to any religion, sect, or other group that conscientiously objected to participation in or support of labor organizations could not be required to join or financially support a union as a condition of employment
- Stated that these amendments superseded all state labor laws that were previously applicable to non-governmental health care provider organizations.

The Congressional intent of the 1975 Taft-Hartley amendments appeared to be to:

- Direct priority attention of the NLRB to labor disputes and unfair labor practice charges in health care
- Make it possible in work stoppage situations to transfer patients to other institutions without the risk of secondary strikes or boycotts
- Reaffirm the NLRB's definitions of supervisors among professional employees in health care institutions
- Keep the number of bargaining units—that is, separate union membership collectives—in the same organization to a practical minimum.

Nevertheless, in the late 1980s the NLRB moved toward greater proliferation of bargaining units. The Board's rule-making authority came under legal challenge, but in April 1991 the United States Supreme Court found in favor of the NLRB, and the new unit designations, first proposed in September 1988 and reaffirmed in March 1989, became permanent. As a result, it is possible for there to be as many as eight bargaining units—that is, eight separate unions—in any acute care hospital regardless of its size. The eight possible units are:

- Registered nurses
- Physicians
- Other professionals
- Technical employees
- Skilled maintenance employees
- Business office clerical employees
- Security guards
- Other non-professional employees.

THE DEPARTMENT MANAGER'S ROLE

If there is no union present and no immediate prospect of one arriving, the average department manager will likely have little concern about unions. However, a union organizing situation can occur at any time; thus, the manager should have some basic knowledge of how a union gets into the organization and how it operates once it is in place.

Before a Union Appears

By far the best way a manager can prevent union organizing is to create and maintain a work environment in which employees feel no need for a union. The appropriate work environment will include:

- A caring management group practicing the belief that satisfied employees are the best producers, that thorough and open communication is essential, and that one of the most important functions of a manager is *listening* to employees. The astute department manager will be aware of one fact of organizational life that every union organizer counts on: If it seems that no one in the organization is listening to them, employees will turn to someone who *will* listen to them.
- Clear, reasonable, and well-communicated work rules and personnel policies, consistently applied to all employees.
- Top management's treatment of first-line supervisors and middle managers as full-fledged members of management. As noted, it

is a grave error to assume that all supervisors are automatically pro-management and anti-union.

- Implementation of major changes only following ample notice and thorough explanation.
- Ongoing communication keeping employees advised of the organization's status and especially its financial position.
- Conveying to employees the honest belief that they and management together can do a better job of serving the organization's customers without the intervention of an outside third party.

Early Organizing Signs and Concerns

On occasion a union bent on organizing the employees of a particular facility may be open and visible about what they are doing right from the start. More often than not, however, a union's initial forays into an organization will be surreptitious. It is not uncommon for a union to quietly test its organizing strength by sounding out the employees regarding the likelihood that they can muster a sufficient level of support to bring the union into the organization. An organizing drive can become costly for the union, so it is not at all unusual for the organizers to quietly scope out conditions and estimate their chances of success before committing their visible presence.

A union will sometimes target a facility for organizing based on a plan they are pursuing to organize employees at most facilities in a particular geographic area. However, it is also common for a facility to be targeted for organizing because a number of employees have asked the union to do so. Even though a few employees have asked the union to organize, however, before holding a representation election, the union will still scope out the facility in an attempt to assess whether the overall climate is favorable.

The first-line managers are—or should be—the first line of defense in a union organizing situation. They are in the best position to be the eyes and ears of management before and during an organizing campaign, and they are best positioned to serve as an effective liaison between the ranks and higher management. By and large, the employees are likely to view the entire organization the way they view their own manager. If the department manager—the single member of management the employees in the department know personally—is seen as cold, indifferent, or uncaring, so too may the entire organization be seen.

Security, always an important issue in a health care organization, takes on added importance when a union is attempting to organize employees or is preparing to do so. Health care organizations, and especially hospitals, can be busy places with a great many people—patients, families, visitors, employees, vendors, and others—moving in and out during the course of a day. Without proper, visible means of identifying who is who at any given time, and without effective visitor control, the average hospital is little more secure than any public gathering place.

When a union is scoping out a facility, organizers commonly enter the facility and "hang out" in the places where employees congregate, such as the cafeteria or snack bar. The organizers can often do this easily unless there is strict visitor control. As outsiders who have no legitimate business in the facility, external organizers can legally be kept out of the building and off the grounds, allowed to come no closer than the public sidewalk. Failing the ability to successfully "infiltrate" the building to talk with employees, external organizers will often visit the outside spots frequented by employees and will sometimes even host off-site informational meetings to which employees are invited.

In addition to testing the interest of employees, organizers will be looking and listening for certain other indications of unrest. They are usually especially interested in identifying problem departments, areas of high turnover and employee dissatisfaction, and particular managers who are disliked for their harsh, authoritarian, or arbitrary treatment of employees. The organizers also look for "martyrs," so-called victims of the system who have supposedly been dealt with unjustly.

Wages, benefits, and other tangibles will almost always receive some mention from the very beginning of union activity, but rarely are these the real drivers that push employees toward a union. Regardless of what sparks employee interest in a union, however, when—or if—the issues ever reach the bargaining table you can rest assured they will be mostly economic issues. A union can demand, and conceivably get, pay and benefits. However, much of what may have been lacking that drove employees toward the union—respect, inclusion, open and honest communication—is sufficiently intangible that it cannot be acquired by contractual demand.

Ask a number of first-line managers to describe the earliest stages of union organizing and chances are many of them will say that the first indication of activity is people passing out union literature on the sidewalks around the facility and at the employee parking entrances. Chances are, however, that once the leaflet distributors show up, the union may have already spent several weeks scoping out the facility and assessing its chances. Union representatives may have already been meeting quietly with groups of interested employees, and may even have spent some time quietly circulating within the facility.

So active literature distribution could mean that the union is becoming serious about organizing and is coming out into the open. On the other hand, it could simply be a random one-shot distribution to see whether the information sparks any interest among employees. Such distribution might be part of a "pass-through," occurring when a union visits, for example, all of the hospitals or nursing homes in a particular area on a given day, passing out informational literature. In addition to containing information about the union and what it claims to be able to do for employees, the material distributed usually includes a postcard that employees can use to request additional information or arrange a personal visit.

Often the department manager has no way of determining for certain whether the department's employees are looking into the possibility of a union or if a union is at work scoping out its potential with the employees. However, when there is active interest in organizing, managers may notice some changes in employee behavior. Specifically:

- New or unusual groupings of employees. When people who have never before congregated with each other now seem close, perhaps even secretive, it could mean that they now share a common interest—in a union.
- Employees from other departments visiting employees in the manager's department during breaks and other personal time. These could be internal organizers—employees of the facility who are working toward union representation.
- Small groups of conversing employees who disband and scatter as any member of management approaches.
- A marked increase in detailed questions about specific employee benefits and other conditions of employment, especially demands to know why some benefits are not more generous or why others are not provided.

- Specific disciplinary actions being openly and vocally challenged, and an increasing tendency of the department's employees to question management's decisions.
- Certain employees being excluded from groups of which they were formerly part. These are often employees known to be loyal to the employer and opposed to a union, so they are frequently kept away from union organizing business.
- Certain employees who would formerly talk with the manager who have fallen silent, no longer willing to be seen conversing with management.

After an Election Petition Arrives

After an election petition arrives, management will work with the organization's labor counsel and usually Human Resources to develop a strategy for dealing with the organizing campaign. Department managers must participate in implementing the strategy by actively campaigning against union representation for their employees. All customary methods of employee communication will apply—meetings, individual discussions, question and answer sessions, and probably a significant number of memos, letters, and other written material.

Managers will have been made aware of the legal limitations on their actions during an organizing campaign and that certain inappropriate conduct could have serious consequences—even to the extent of negating the results of an election. A "freedom of speech" provision in the National Labor Relations Act describes the general boundaries of management's conduct during an organizing campaign. Section 8(c) of the Act states:

> The expressing of any views, argument, or opinion, or the dissemination thereof, whether in written, printed, graphic, or visual form, shall not constitute or be evidence of an unfair labor practice under any of the provisions of this Act, if such expression contains no threat of reprisal or force or promise of benefits.[4]

This section guarantees employers and unions the right to actively campaign, within certain limits, during an organizing drive. That is, the union has the right to attempt to sell its position to the employees and convince them to vote for union representation, and the employer has the right to persuade employees that they are better off without the union's presence.

It should always be considered necessary to actively campaign against a union's bid to represent an employee group. Employees are often told what they want to hear and what is known to appeal to them, but most unions are not known for full and frank disclosure of all implications of unionization in that they neglect to mention some of the perceived negatives of membership.

What Managers Can Do

During union organizing efforts, managers are permitted to express opinions or present arguments to employees and discuss the union and the election with them. Managers may discuss the advantages of remaining union-free, for example citing:

- How the organization's wages and benefits compare with the wages and benefits at unionized facilities
- How existing benefits compare with those offered or promised by the union.

It is also permissible to enumerate the disadvantages of union membership, which may include:

- Costly dues
- Loss of income during strikes and other work stoppages
- The possibility of fines and special assessments for union members
- The possibility of being required to serve on picket lines
- The inability to discuss problems directly with management
- The likelihood that the union will demand union-shop provisions, requiring membership as a condition of employment
- The possibility that a strike may disrupt services and endanger patient health and safety.

Concerning a possible upcoming union election, managers are allowed to inform employees that:

- Signing a union authorization card is not a vote for the union, and doing so does not obligate the employee to vote for the union
- A representation election is conducted by secret ballot so that no one will know how an individual voted

- The outcome of a representation election is determined by the majority of the employees who actually vote, and not by a majority of all eligible voters, so it is critically important that all who do not want union representation be certain to vote—because those who do want the union will vote
- Unless it is a relatively rare independent union, a local union is subject to the governance of its international union—so considerable control over the facility can be exerted from some distance
- Labor law allows the organization to permanently replace any employee who goes on strike for economic reasons (that is, a strike not called because of unfair labor practices)
- Despite any promises the organizers may make, no union can force the employer to pay more than it is willing or able to pay.

What Managers Cannot Do

There are a few prohibitions concerning what managers can say and do during union organizing. These can be summarized in the four-point "TIPS" (or, in some quarters, "PITS" or "SPIT") Rule that essentially captures all of the prohibitions in four simply stated precautions. In addressing union organizing, management cannot:

- **T**hreaten
- **I**nterrogate
- **P**romise
- **S**py.

A communication is not protected by the free-speech provisions of the NLRA if it contains any of these four elements. In the way of specific examples, during union organizing management is restrained from:

- Promising that wages and benefits will be improved if the union loses the representation election
- Making promises of pay increases, promotions, or other special favors to individual employees in exchange for opposing the union
- Threatening employees with the likelihood of job losses, demotions, pay cuts, benefits reductions, and such if the union wins
- Transferring employees and changing assignments to isolate union supporters or break up concentrations of pro-union employees

- Threatening to terminate operations if the union wins
- Asking employees how they intend to vote, what they think about the union, who is or is not supporting the union, or any specific question about an individual's relationship with a union
- Questioning prospective employees about past or present union affiliations
- Spying on union meetings or attempting to determine who is attending
- Using a third party to threaten, intimidate, or coerce employees
- Visiting the homes of employees for purposes of campaigning (unions may visit employees' homes, but employers are forbidden to do so).

The managers of the employees who are being targeted for union organization are key players in counter-organizing activities, answering to those who are orchestrating the drive—the facility's labor attorney, Human Resources or labor relations, and Administration.

Sometime after a union has come out into the open about organizing, management may receive an official communication from the union providing a list of internal organizers. These will be employees of the various departments being targeted. Once these individuals have been openly identified, their department managers must become extremely careful in their dealings with them. They must of course be required to observe all the same rules and job requirements of other employees—being internal organizers gives them no special privileges—but since they have declared their organizing status they will be intentionally sensitive to any treatment they might choose to claim is discriminatory. It is highly likely that by officially identifying its internal organizers in this manner, the union is hoping to trap management into committing unfair labor practices.

Some time before the election there may be challenges concerning the composition of the unit and some employees' eligibility to vote. Technically supervisors and managers are not included in union membership (except in some governmental institutions where representation is provided by public employer unions), but there are often legitimate questions about who is employed in a true supervisory capacity. Whether one side or the other wants supervisors included or excluded may hinge on how it is believed these people would vote concerning union membership.

Generally, management will attempt to have supervisory personnel excluded from eligibility; in many instances—for example, units that include registered nurses (RNs) and licensed practical nurses (LPNs) in supervisory or pseudo-supervisory positions—the union will want to include them. When unit composition is challenged, ordinarily the regional office of the National Labor Relations Board will hold a unit-determination hearing to determine whether these "supervisors" fit the definition contained in the National Labor Relations Act, specifically: Do these employees have the authority to hire, transfer, suspend, lay off, recall, promote, discharge, assign, reward or discipline, responsibly direct employees, adjust grievances, *or to recommend such action?* The NLRB will further assess whether the exercise of that authority requires the use of independent judgment and whether the employee holds the authority in the interest of the employer. Both employer and union present their arguments for including or excluding the employees in question, and the NLRB renders a decision that defines the unit's membership.

The activity leading up to a representation election can be frantic and time-consuming for those who are working to keep the facility union-free. Although there are numerous rules to be observed on both sides of the process, there is a single overriding concern that drives both management and the union: the need to win. Frequently each side will be watching the other carefully for signs of irregularities, and it is not unusual for charges of improper conduct to fly back and forth.

When the actual day of the election arrives, the rules change. Managers may continue to speak with employees individually and pass out printed information, but must now avoid holding group meetings on work time where employees are obliged to hear the employer's anti-union message. It is the position of the NLRB that much of that final day before votes are cast should belong to the employees, as free from interference as possible. The safest approach for management is to refrain from active campaigning on the day of the election, and perhaps limit the involvement of managers on this day to responding to questions that employees may ask.

After voting occurs, even though the count will usually be available immediately, there is ordinarily a period of days before the NLRB will certify the results of the election and make them official. A simple majority of those voting will determine the outcome unless a sufficient number of votes are challenged to throw the outcome into question. The election will have been monitored by a number of employees on behalf of both sides, and if anyone's voting eligibility appears questionable to the monitors, the person's vote may be challenged. Challenged votes become a critical concern only if they would make a difference in the outcome. For example, if the results of an election are Union-50; No Union-54; Challenged-6, the challenged votes could make a difference in who wins and who loses, so the regional NLRB has more work to do. But if the election results are Union-58; No Union-46; Challenged-6, the outcome is established because even if all of the challenged votes went to No Union the total would still not change the outcome.

Should the union lose the election, it can try again after one year has passed. NLRB rules require a lapse of at least one year before another election can be held involving the same unit of employees. It perhaps strikes many in management as unfair that a union attempting to organize a particular group can theoretically lose year after year for several years before finally getting in, while the employer need lose but once to have the union there forever for all practical purposes.

Immediately after the election the department manager may have some work to do in helping put the immediate past, the campaign, and the possible hard feelings generated behind all concerned and get on with the business of running the institution. Regardless of the outcome of the election, the end of campaign activity will usually provide welcome relief for the manager, who can then resume work at a more reasonable pace.

Dealing with a Union Day-to-Day

If the employees have chosen union representation, all channels of employee communication must still be kept open to the fullest possible extent. This is no time for the manager to back off simply because there are now union representatives regularly talking with employees. The department manager must learn the legal requirements of dealing with a union and must develop a complete understanding of the collective bargaining agreement—that is, the contract—that is negotiated.

Often one of the first contract provisions negotiated is that calling for a union shop; that is, a provision stating that new employees entering the covered unit are required to join the union within a given period of time—30, 60, or 90 days are common time frames—as a condition of continued employment. This is an extremely important provision to the union, the leadership of which understandably wants dues from all persons who will benefit from their negotiations.

Some department managers may find that coexistence with a union brings a certain predictability to relationships with employees. Rules will now be in place governing many activities that may formerly have depended on supervisory decision-making. For example, where previously a manager may have had to wrestle with a specific employee complaint and determine what could be done to resolve it, there may now be a formal grievance procedure that must be followed. The manager might not care much for the process or the outcomes it generates, but this manager no longer has to come up with a solution. As another example, the union contract may contain a specific protocol for assigning overtime; this relieves the manager of any responsibility for decisions about overtime since he or she is required to simply follow the protocol. Some department managers find that they prefer this sort of predictability.

For the most part, the department manager should be able to adjust to existing with a union. The union's presence may not be the manager's preference. Even though some facets of day-to-day functioning will become more predictable, in a number of ways the union will make life more difficult. There will be additional channels of communication to maintain, and the manager had best never forget that this union—this third party now present in every relationship—has its own agenda separate from the needs of both its members and management.

DECERTIFICATION

As initially passed, the National Labor Relations Act strongly favored unions and took considerable steps to protect employees from the abuses of employers. In 1947 the Labor Management Reporting Act (Taft-Hartley), in amending the NLRA, took a more balanced approach to protecting the rights of individual employees from abuse by both employers and unions. Taft-Hartley made it possible for employees to get out from under a union that seemed to no longer serve their purposes or be acting in their best interests. This change allowed employees to remove a union when its leaders failed to meet membership expectations. Taft-Hartley permitted decertifications of bargaining units for the first time. Decertifications are not common, but they do occur now and then.

A petition asking for decertification cannot be filed within what is referred to as the union's "certification year." A newly chosen union is given this initial year to negotiate a contract and demonstrate what it can do for its members. Whether for initial choosing of a union or for decertification, there can be only one representation election in a particular bargaining unit within a 12-month period.

First and foremost for the department manager to be aware of concerning a decertification is that management cannot in any way be involved in initiating a move toward decertification. Concerning decertification, managers generally cannot:

- Volunteer information to employees about how decertification can be accomplished
- Tell employees they would probably be treated better without the union present
- Suggest that employees generate a petition to decertify the union
- Behave in a manner that is intended to encourage employees to pursue the decertification process.

Essentially all that management is legally permitted to do during the initiation stage of decertification is to respond to employees' questions about decertification. Doing so cannot include any encouragement to pursue decertification or any unsolicited advice on how to go about doing so.

Should a decertification effort reach the petition stage, the employer can still do little more than respond to employees' questions. At this stage, however, some responses can be more specific and essentially more helpful. For instance, management can direct employees to the appropriate authorities at the National Labor Relations Board and can provide additional information about the decertification process as long as doing so is in direct response to employee inquiries. However, this is really assistance at a minimal level when we consider that management is still forbidden to:

- Help with the wording of the petition, or allow the petition to be transmitted on the organization's letterhead
- Allow employees to solicit petition signatures during working hours, or to provide management space for signing to occur
- Provide time off for an employee to file the petition.

Once a decertification petition is filed and a decertification election campaign officially begins, management can take additional actions subject to two important limitations: management may not interfere with the employees' right to choose between decertification or not, and management's behavior must be free from promises and threats (i.e., the "TIPS" rule) that could upset the conditions under which employees are to choose. Management is allowed to express its views about whether the union should be present as long as these views do not include direct or implied threats of reprisals for retaining the union or promises of rewards for removing the union. For example, management cannot suggest that a wage increase will follow if the union is decertified or that certain benefits will have to be curtailed should the union remain in place. At this stage of the decertification campaign, management may:

- Communicate its views to employees by letter
- Give employees comparisons of wages and benefits of union and non-union workers
- Hold meetings with employees, provided that employee attendance is voluntary.

Discussion Points

1. Explain why it appears that unionization within health care is increasing while union membership in the total work force continues to decline. Include your assessment of why unions are apparently targeting health care.
2. Define an *unfair labor practice* and provide three or four examples.
3. Discuss why can it be said that the majority of union elections are won or lost by management long before the union ever shows up.
4. If it is indeed usually non-economic issues that drive employees to become organized, consider why very nearly all of the demands that cross the bargaining table have dollar signs attached to them.
5. Explain why it is advisable to have in place a comprehensive policy governing solicitation and the posting of information

on the premises before any signs of active union organizing appear.

6. Explain why it is considerably more difficult to get a union out through decertification than it is to have a union come into the organization.

7. Provide two specific examples of behavior that represent each of the four prohibitions on management conduct during union organizing: threatening, interrogating, promising, and spying.

8. Two of your employees stop you in the middle of a busy corridor in the facility, and one of them says: "We want to talk to you about this union stuff that's going around. Now." Explain how will you respond and what you will do.

9. As a department manager over unionized employees, consider whether you believe it would be preferable to have your employees in a specifically dedicated bargaining unit (such as registered nurses only, security officers only, etc.) or a "wall-to-wall" unit (one that includes employees in all capacities). Why?

10. Discuss the advantages and disadvantages to the manager of working day-to-day with a union contract.

11. Explain why the distribution of union literature to employees arriving or departing work is frequently assumed to be the first stage of active union organizing.

12. Your organization is experiencing a union organizing campaign. Draft a brief (two- or three-paragraph) speech to give to your employees at a staff meeting to encourage them to think carefully about favoring union membership, keeping your comments strictly legal.

13. You manage a department of unionized professionals who have become disillusioned with their union. Three of your employees ask you to help them get their union decertified. Discuss what you can do for them.

14. It has been repeatedly stated that the first-line manager is the essential communicating link with rank-and-file employees in an organizing situation. Consider why, then, so many first-line managers appear unwilling to speak up or become involved when a union is actively organizing.

15. Identify the key differences between health care and non-health industries in the manner in which work stoppages may be conducted.

NOTES

[1]Knight Ridder News Service, "Unions Set Sights on High-Tech Workers," *Democrat & Chronicle*, Rochester NY, September 20, 2000.

[2]The Associated Press, "Stressed Nurses Striking More," *Democrat & Chronicle*, Rochester NY, June 1, 2001.

[3]Ibid.

[4]29 U.S.C. Section 158(c) (1984).

CHAPTER 16

The Manager's Role in Employee Training

This chapter—

- Discusses the importance of training and development as a continuing activity
- Outlines the essential role of the department manager as a teacher
- Stresses the importance of new-employee orientation at the department level
- Presents principles applicable in addressing staff training and development needs
- Addresses cross-training as a means for improving employee capability and departmental effectiveness
- Suggests how to and also how not to approach on-the-job training
- Outlines a suggested approach to employee mentoring
- Stresses the importance of developing potential managers among the staff
- Suggests how Human Resources can help the manager meet the department's training needs.

THE KEY ROLE OF TRAINING AND DEVELOPMENT

Executive management in most health care institutions can be counted on to praise the value of continuing education and to vocalize its support for this supposedly essential activity. Unfortunately, however, a significant percentage of executive management can also be counted on to place education on the chopping block when money gets tight and expenses must be reduced. This is perhaps at least partly due to the difficulty of pinpointing cost savings that can be attributed to education. Most individuals in management perhaps know intuitively, or at least believe, that education ultimately saves money. The problem is that there is no reliable way of measuring the results of education in terms of cost-benefit analysis, so education is too readily viewed as money going out with nothing tangible coming in.

As important as training and development is to every department, in many instances it receives scant attention from department management. It is perhaps not sufficient to simply remind department managers that they all have a responsibility for employee development. Rather, perhaps they should be encouraged to view training and development as an important part of the means of keeping valuable employees interested and challenged.

It has been well-established in recent decades that the factors that truly motivate employees are found primarily in the work itself, and among the strongest motivating factors are the opportunity to do interesting and challenging work and the opportunity to learn and grow. Not all employees are so motivated, but the better performers usually are, and it is the better performers who are more likely to leave for greener pastures in search of more interesting and challenging work and greater opportunity overall. One way for the department manager to increase the chances of retaining the better employees is through visible support of training and development.

It has often been said that if we seem to be standing still, then we are actually going backward. This in part describes a department that places no emphasis on training and development. With change constantly occurring on the technological, economic, legislative, financial, and social fronts, no one in health care can afford to stand still. A certain amount of forward progress is necessary simply to remain abreast of change. Therefore, maintaining or improving the abilities of staff must be an ongoing effort. Continuing education is essential.

THE MANAGER'S ROLE IN EMPLOYEE TRAINING

Under the blanket heading of *training* we include the entire range of employee development activities, from providing orientation for new employees to assisting employees in moving up into management. Employee development is—or should be—one of the most important aspects of a department manager's role.

As a department manager, you likely have greater depth and breadth of technical knowledge and expertise in the function you manage than is found anywhere else in the organization. Chances are you were educated in the primary field in which you work, and in addition to that formal education you have the advantage of the practical education you have acquired through work. Therefore, you are a primary resource for information about your department and the work it performs. All of this places you, the department manager, in the best of all possible positions for passing your knowledge and expertise along to others. Moreover, as department manager you have the responsibility for maintaining and improving the capability and competence of your staff.

The importance of continuing education and training is underscored by the extent to which the various accreditation and regulatory agencies assess training activities during their periodic surveys. Another measure of this importance is these agencies' requirements for many health care practitioners to provide evidence of a certain amount of continuing education each year to maintain their professional licensure.

From the manager's perspective, teaching should be an integral part of the management role. Certainly teaching is an essential part of proper delegation. Unfortunately, employee instruction—teaching the person to do the job that he or she has been assigned to perform—is one of the weaker parts of delegation as practiced, a weakness that often leads to delegation failure.

Orientation: Getting Them Started Right

Each department manager should have a new-employee orientation plan for the department. This of course is not news to managers in nursing and a number of other clinical disciplines, since orientation plans are required by accreditation and regulation.

The organization will usually provide a general new-employee orientation that addresses matters common to all departments. Ordinarily provided by Human Resources, or perhaps by a separate education department, the general orientation will address such matters as the organization's structure and leadership, employee benefits, the performance appraisal process, the organization's dress code, employee parking, facility security, infection control and universal precautions, employee health services and other forms of assistance such as the employee assistance program (EAP), employee work rules, and generally applicable policies.

There is no need to duplicate any of the general orientation in the department orientation. Rather, the department orientation should be just that—an introduction to the people in the department and to the physical area, equipment, processes, and special department policies, as well as on-the-job guidance in getting started doing the work.

One of the most inappropriate ways of treating a new employee, even an experienced person who supposedly knows the activity or occupation hands-down, is to simply turn this person loose to make his or her own way. Even the experienced and well-educated new employee needs guidance concerning the variations specific to this department in this organization, as well as some extra attention for the time required for the new and perhaps strange to start to become familiar.

As part of a new employee's departmental orientation, it may help to consider mentoring—pairing a new employee with an experienced person who can provide guidance through the new person's first few days or weeks as necessary. Mentoring offers a valuable two-fold benefit: It provides a personally guided orientation for the newcomer, and it is an opportunity for further development on the part of the experienced employee, the mentor.

Training for Correcting Performance Problems

We have said that training ought to be a manager's priority. Obviously, however, it is not the manager's top priority; that honor goes to running the department to get out the work expected of the department. Nevertheless, training is essential, especially training employees in new or revised work procedures and training employees to correct performance problems.

In assessing how well employees are doing on the job, the manager will be continually comparing observed performance with expected performance. The manager may need to be very much the teacher when it comes to helping employees correct performance problems (see Chapter 9, The Health Care Manager and Employee Problems). When an employee exhibits performance problems that command the manager's attention, it is always appropriate for the manager to consider whether he or she is doing all that can reasonably be done to help this employee succeed. Any number of employees fail at their jobs not because they were not smart enough to succeed or because they simply could not do the work, but rather because they were inappropriately trained, insufficiently oriented, or inadequately supported.

On occasion it may be necessary to make some particular kind of education or training a condition of continued employment. For example, an individual whose telephone manner has elicited many complaints may be required to complete a program in telephone etiquette, or one whose job requires writing but who has experienced problems with written grammar may be required to take a remedial English program.

Looking at Departmental Learning Needs

If a variety of learning needs seem to present themselves throughout the department, it might be helpful to conduct a basic learning-needs analysis. One approach to a learning-needs analysis consists of making a simple chart for each job description in the department, with perhaps columns indicating the principal skills required and rows listing the employees who work to that job description. It becomes a matter of assessing each employee in terms of whether his or her skills are adequate to meet normal job expectations in each skill category. Each assessment that falls short of normal expectations indicates a learning need; this approach helps the manager focus training activities on areas of greatest need. In addition to the manager's assessment, noticeable performance problems indicate areas of need, as do tendencies toward repetitive errors or chronic complaints by customers, coworkers, and others.

The manager's initial consideration in expressing any training need for any employee should be the articulation of an objective or objectives. The learner must initially know where it is that he or she must be going; once this is determined, the learner and the manager can proceed with their consideration of how to get there.

Always, the learner's motivation is a key to the eventual success of the training, and the manager must always be prepared to help the employee answer one particular question about what he or she is being asked to learn: "What's in it for me?" In correcting a severe performance problem, the answer may be as basic as "You get to remain employed." But there are numerous other possible answers, such as: "You get to learn something that may eventually help get you promoted"; "You get more variety in your work"; and "You get to do something more challenging than what you've been doing."

Employee Training within the Department

Following are a few principles that may assist the department manager in addressing staff training and development needs:

- Employees learn better when they become actually involved in the process, so the more training can be hands-on, learn-while-doing, the more likely it is to be successful.
- Employees will more quickly and accurately absorb material that applies to their daily work rather than having to learn material they see as irrelevant; thus, in-department employee training should be practical and immediately applicable rather than theoretical.
- Most employees will accept new ideas more readily if these ideas support their previous beliefs, so new material, new techniques, and new processes are best presented within the context of the department's mission. For example, "We're still here to do (this) for the patient, but now it can be done more quickly and at lower cost."
- Some employees learn best when allowed to pursue their own areas of interest or need at their own rate. For these employees the manager must provide clear expectations, necessary information and materials, and perhaps general guidance.
- Many employees need to be encouraged to find learning pleasant. To some employees the possibility of education of any kind essentially means "going back to school," which leaves them automatically resistant. Again, they must be shown what's in it for them.
- All employees who are expected to learn something deserve to know *why* they are learning, and all should be advised of specific goals and objectives.

Cross-Training for Efficiency

The department manager who supervises employees who work in roughly comparable positions as far as job grade and pay scale are concerned usually has the opportunity to implement cross-training. Say, for example, a business office manager has six clerical-level employees who are assigned two each in three capacities: cashier, file clerk, and data entry operator. These three jobs reside in the same pay grade. As long as these six people simply do their own jobs all of the time, the department has limited flexibility. If one cashier is on vacation and the other is taken ill, there are no trained cashiers available; likewise, if one data entry operator is gone for two weeks and the other fails to keep up with the total demand, data entry falls behind. But if all six people are capable of doing all three jobs, employees can be moved around as needed. Resources can be shifted about as workloads or backlogs demand, and any of the six people is capable of covering for any of the others as necessary.

All it takes to gain this type of flexibility is to train the six employees in each others' jobs. Certainly there is some work involved in doing so, but since each of the six is skilled in one of the jobs, for each job there are two people who are capable of doing most of the training of the other four with no more involvement of the manager than general guidance. This training will ultimately prove well worth the time and effort. The department stands to gain considerable flexibility in addressing backlogs and covering for vacations and illnesses, and the individuals gain greater interest and challenge associated with their work through greater task variety.

On-the-Job Training

On-the-job training is appropriate under many circumstances, and for some learning needs it may be the best available approach—if it is pursued properly. Much on-the-job training is best accomplished under the direct supervision of the department manager or under the direct guidance of an experienced employee. The employee being trained on the job receives step-by-step instructions on how to accomplish a task while actually performing the task. After the employee performs the task a sufficient number of times under this direct guidance, the instructor may then reduce or eliminate the verbal guidance and simply watch the employee until assured that the activity is being performed satisfactorily. Thus assured, the instructor may further withdraw to a position of being readily available to answer questions.

What on-the-job training is decidedly *not* is turning the employee loose to learn by trial and error with only a rough idea of expected results. However, this is precisely what it becomes in many instances, most often when the manager fancies himself or herself too busy to address training properly or, perhaps even worse, adopts an attitude that implies: "Once I had to figure this out for myself, so now it's your turn." Unfortunately, what some managers describe as on-the-job training is exactly what on-the-job training is not: placing an employee on the job with minimal preparation and letting the person work through the problems and frustrations alone.

Improper on-the-job training can of course be dangerous and even destructive; even if there are no critical quality implications to a given task, there are clearly negative potential results of self-training. The employee may learn to perform the task in a highly inefficient manner, building inappropriate work habits that will become deeply ingrained and difficult to correct. It is far better for the manager to ensure that the proper amount of time and attention are devoted at the start of the learning process so that on-the-job training can succeed as intended.

Another commonly encountered approach to training, or at least to the satisfaction of annual in-service education requirements, is the "reading file" approach to accomplishing the staff's annual review of certain documents as required by accreditation or regulation. A reading package is circulated throughout the staff with instructions for each recipient to review the documents as required, check off to indicate they have done so, and pass the material to the next person. This is the loosest and undoubtedly the weakest approach to "training" of any kind, since there is no way short of questioning each recipient in detail to ensure that the material has been read and absorbed.

It has repeatedly been established that most people recall a certain portion of information they hear, a somewhat greater portion of what they both see and hear, and an even greater portion of what they see, hear, and do. This suggests that some of the most effective job-related training includes a combination of lecture, demonstration, and hands-on practice. To be somewhat more specific (while rounding some figures that are arguably approximations only), research on learning processes has shown that the majority of people will remember:

- 10 percent of what they read
- 20 percent of what they hear
- 30 percent of what they see
- 50 percent of what they see and hear
- 80 percent of what they say
- 90 percent of what they say as they do.

Two strong suggestions for training activities are implicit in these research claims. First, appealing to multiple senses increases the likelihood of learning. This is why personal reading alone can be the least effective way of learning, and why lecture alone is not a great deal better; when multiple senses are applied simultaneously, the chances of learning increase accordingly. Second, spaced repetition—the same material repeated after a lapse of time, and perhaps presented in varying forms—can be highly effective in ensuring that the material will be retained.

EFFECTIVE MENTORING

Mentoring can be most effective if it is made official. It need not take place within the context of a formal program, but it should at least be acknowledged as an actively used employee development technique rather than simply an *ad hoc* practice whereby people might happen to link up with each other. The extent of the formality required is no more than the following:

- The newer employee (mentee) and experienced employee (mentor) are intentionally brought together by the department manager.
- Three parties—mentee, mentor, and manager—agree on the objectives of the relationship, specifying what the mentee is expected to learn.
- The department manager remains close enough to the process to be able to evaluate both mentee and mentor during and after the mentoring period.

By officially addressing mentoring as a means of employee development, the organization sends a strong message to all employees concerning its commitment to employee development. Although mentoring is one of the least costly development tools available, it can be extremely effective, and its visible use plainly says that the organization cares about the development of its people.

For a newer employee, a mentor can be a valuable facilitator, sounding board, and source of advice and guidance. The mentor also can benefit as well. Mentoring can provide a sense of fulfillment and satisfaction, especially for a senior employee who is in need of additional challenge and who could benefit from more interesting work experiences. Mentoring helps the mentors further refine their skills and keep them sharp.

The employee most likely to realize significant benefit from a mentoring relationship is one who:

- Demonstrates an evident willingness to learn, is proactive in expressing this willingness, and is obviously ambitious and enthusiastic

- Seems able to assume full responsibility for his or her own growth and development
- Demonstrates receptiveness to coaching and constructive feedback and the ability to change behavior based on positive experiences.

The experienced employee who is considered for mentoring responsibilities should be one who:

- Is willing to serve voluntarily (no mentor should ever be unilaterally assigned or forced to serve) and give the undertaking the time and energy it requires
- Possesses sufficient knowledge and expertise in the mentee's areas of responsibility
- Possesses strong interpersonal skills (specifically, is patient, supportive, friendly, and an effective listener)
- Demonstrates an interest in the development of others.

DEVELOPING POTENTIAL MANAGERS

It should be considered an essential part of every manager's responsibility to help in identifying and developing new managers, and certainly in identifying and developing one or more potential successors. This latter need represents an area where many managers fall short.

The development of potential successors is of course closely associated with the practice of proper delegation, which is the primary means by which this development proceeds. This is an area of concern into which some managers seem unwilling to proceed. Some are insecure in their position and fear the competition provided by intelligent, up-and-coming subordinates. Or perhaps the manager simply does not think appreciably beyond the present, and is thus ill prepared to imagine being moved up or out or becoming incapacitated and no longer able to function in that position.

Often in-department development of a potential new manager does not occur simply because it requires the sort of serious delegation that takes time and planning on the part of the department manager, and there never seems to be quite enough time to get it done. Also, such development requires delegation of tasks of increasing responsibility—tasks that are often sufficiently appealing or "important" that the manager retains them personally rather than giving them up to a subordinate.

At the very least, having a potential successor in the process of development means that the department manager usually has readily available coverage for vacations and illness as necessary. No one person is absolutely indispensable, but the loss or absence of a group's leader when there is no ready back-up can create significant inefficiency and inconvenience.

The department manager who may perhaps entertain ambitions about advancing higher in the organization had best take seriously the need to develop a potential successor. Higher management will often look closely at a manager's track record at delegating, and especially at whether that manager has one or more capable successors in the wings. Enlightened higher management may well conclude that a department manager who has paid no attention to developing a potential successor shows little strength in delegation, a skill that becomes increasingly important as one moves up the chain of command. Also, those above in the hierarchy may not be willing to promote the department manager if doing so means conducting an external search for a successor or promoting an untried insider.

No manager wants to lose the department's better employees. However, some of them are going to be lost regardless of what the manager does. The manager who puts time and effort into developing potential successors may see many of them eventually lost to other departments or other organizations as they take advantage of opportunities to advance their careers. But these employees are fully as likely to be lost if they are not subject to development; in all likelihood some of them will be lost even sooner if they remain unchallenged in their jobs. Therefore the department manager had best take full advantage of the talents that are available in the group by delegating to the better and more willing employees and helping them develop.

Only extremely rarely does a department manager have anything to fear from a subordinate who is encouraged to develop and grow and learn some aspects of the manager's job. In fact, having one or two sharp, up-and-coming employees right behind him or her could be just what the department manager needs to remain sharp and to keep growing as a manager.

HOW HUMAN RESOURCES CAN HELP

It is customary for the organization's general new-employee orientation to be presented or at least coordinated by Human Resources.

As far as this orientation is concerned, ordinarily all the department manager has to do is ensure that each new employee attends. However, some department managers have to be reminded of the necessity for all employees to attend the orientation. Some of these new employees may be filling positions that have been empty for some time and the department may be behind in its work, so an occasional manager may decide that the new employee cannot be spared for the few hours that orientation requires. There is sometimes a tendency to regard orientation as "another Human Resources thing" that intrudes on the manager's ability to run a department. In most instances, however, a general orientation to the organization includes topics that are required by accreditation and regulation, so orientation is partly a response to external requirements and partly a service performed to get new employees pointed in the proper direction.

Beyond ensuring that new employees attend general orientation, it is the manager's responsibility to be aware of training needs and to either attend to them or refer them as necessary. In addressing issues of employee training and development, the department manager should expect Human Resources to:

- Work with the manager in diagnosing particular problems and determining the kinds of training or education that might be helpful
- Provide certain kinds of needed training directly by Human Resources staff
- Secure the involvement of other in-house training expertise as needed to address specific needs
- Identify external sources of specifically required training and determine how these sources are accessed
- Guide employees in using the organization's tuition assistance program when appropriate.

Training needs should be addressed on a continuing basis, both to (1) assess present circumstances to determine the skills and attitudes that need to be adopted or improved to meet current needs, and (2) attempt to determine future needs based on what trends appear to be coming during the next one or two years. Information for judging training needs can be gathered in a variety of ways, including questionnaires completed by both managers and employees, focus group discussions, individual interviews of managers and employees, and exit interviews at which departing employees are asked for their opinions concerning developmental needs. Those topics that surface more frequently and most strongly will merit closer scrutiny as potential program topics.

Human Resources can contribute information relevant to determining training and development needs from:

- Direct contact with people on the job, both managers and rank-and-file employees
- Reviews of various records accessible by HR, including performance appraisals, performance improvement records, and disciplinary actions
- Trends evident in the health care industry
- Insights into what is current or coming in human resources development in health care.

In guiding any training and development activity, Human Resources will likely recommend:

- Involving both managers and employees in preparing training agendas and determining program content
- Starting, if at all possible, with needs the employees appear to be the most strongly motivated to address
- Focusing on present jobs and present needs first, then looking to the future
- Focusing primarily on behavior, in the belief that if skills are appropriately implanted or modified then the proper attitudes will follow
- Using on-the-job experiential learning to the maximum extent practical, supplemented from other sources.

In assessing training efforts after the fact, Human Resources will attempt to determine:

- Whether the needs assessments that were done were correct
- Whether targeted skills have been learned and incorporated in behavior
- Whether attitudes appear to have been modified
- What has been learned, and how this assessment of results can feed into the next cycle of training.

Discussion Points

1. Consider why training and development opportunities are important to certain employees but apparently not to others. To which employees do they appear most important?
2. Discuss why it is important for the training and development *opportunity* to be available even if not many take advantage of it.
3. Explain why in-service or on-the-job education must of necessity be *continuing*.
4. Explain in some detail why you believe education is usually one of the first line items to be reduced or eliminated when it becomes necessary to cut budgets.
5. List several activities that you could engage in as a department manager to continue involving your employees in education with little or no direct budgetary impact.
6. Using either an actual or a hypothetical department having three or four roughly comparable positions, describe how you would implement a program of cross-training among the employees.
7. Discuss how the department manager's role as an instructor, teacher, or mentor relates to his or her role in effective delegation.
8. Explain why should it be considered important for the department manager who plans on remaining in place for as long as practical to nevertheless be developing one or two capable employees as potential successors.
9. It is frequently claimed that it is difficult if not impossible to quantify the cost effectiveness of education. Discuss whether or not you believe this to be true.
10. Describe the advantages of using capable senior employees as mentors or trainers for newer employees.

CHAPTER 17

Iceberg Tips: Compensation, Benefits, and Other Concerns

This chapter—

- Describes Human Resources' role and the department manager's involvement in compensation
- Provides an overview of HR's and the department manager's roles regarding benefits
- Discusses the department manager's occasional role concerning statutory benefits (e.g., worker's compensation, short-term disability)
- Contrasts the manager's role in the employment process with what occurs behind the scenes in Human Resources
- Describes what transpires behind the scenes in Human Resources concerning performance appraisal
- Offers summary guidelines for the manager who becomes involved in legal action
- Provides an overview of Human Resources' involvement in external agency investigations, highlighting the manager's likely involvements.

Only a limited portion of many Human Resources activities is visible to the department manager. The activities discussed in this chapter are hidden in the sense that most of what occurs with them happens within Human Resources and elsewhere other than the department manager's sphere of responsibility. This chapter is intended to provide the department manager with a basic understanding of what occurs beneath the surface of these "iceberg tips."

COMPENSATION

One of Human Resources' primary responsibilities is to maintain the organization's compensation structure. HR ordinarily remains current with compensation levels in the health care industry and the local labor market. On some predetermined basis, usually annually, Human Resources will be expected to make recommendations for changes in compensation that will likely go before the organization's board of directors for consideration. The annual compensation recommendations may consist of:

- Suggested timing of compensation changes and the rationale for the suggested distribution of increases
- Proposed wage increases to be applied either to all employees or to employees in specific occupations
- Proposed changes in the compensation scales (i.e., the stated pay ranges for all of the organization's job categories)
- The basis for the compensation changes being proposed (usually anchored in prevailing industry or area compensation practices).

Knowing the Compensation System

For the purpose of addressing compensation questions for employees, the department manager will ordinarily be expected to know:

- How pay increases are related to performance (if such is the system), and generally the level of performance (as reflected in performance appraisal scores) required for receiving merit-based increases
- The differences between merit pay increases and increases achieved through pay-scale movement (or supposed "cost-of-living" increases)
- When merit increases or scale increases can usually be expected to occur
- How and when other kinds of pay increases, specifically probationary increases (if the system provides for such), are granted.

The manager should also be conversant with the current pay scales for all positions in the department, and should maintain current pay-scale data for reference. When pay scales are changed, Human Resources supplies up-to-date published pay scales to the department managers. The manager ordinarily requires current pay-scale information in addressing certain employee questions and for other related reasons, but the dissemination of this information should be selective, based on need to know or right to know.

Any individual employee can be considered as having the right to know his or her pay scale—expressed, perhaps, as hourly rate minimum, maximum, and possibly midpoint—as well as his or her own actual rate of pay. However, no individual employee is entitled to know other employees' pay scales or any other individual employee's rate of pay, so the department manager has responsibility for safeguarding this aspect of employee privacy.

When Compensation Challenges Arise

The department manager is often the initial target for challenges to the compensation system raised by employees. Some individual employees seem frequently compelled to challenge their rates of pay with claims of inequities arising from comparison of what they are paid with what certain others who are similarly situated (be it according to occupation, job title, or other comparative means) are paid for performing essentially the same or comparable work.

The department manager should recognize several responsibilities related to possible pay inequities. First, the manager should know enough about the pay level of each person in the department to be able to recognize pay inequities within the group when they surface. The manager who has a small group of employees may be well aware of how these people stack up against each other in terms of pay, so in a relatively small group a substantial pay inequity usually will not occur. But in a larger department, with the cumulative effects of several years' hiring at differing levels as well as merit, probationary, and annual increases occurring, the occasional inequity may remain hidden until some employee brings it to the fore. When this occurs, the manager should do some preliminary research concerning the inequity, and, if warranted, bring it to Human Resources for further analysis and possibly a recommendation for correction.

The manager's other responsibility with regard to supposed pay inequities is to work with Human Resources when the challenges involve claims of underpayment in comparison with what persons of comparable skills are supposedly receiving at other local facilities. Employees will sometimes approach the department manager with such challenges looking for the manager's support and advocacy—wanting the manager to champion their cause and seek to have one or more pay scales increased and corresponding pay raises granted for individuals.

Although it is a natural inclination for a conscientious and caring manager to advocate for the department's employees at various times, when it comes to claims of pay inequity with other organizations it is best to involve Human Resources before agreeing to take on the employee's cause. Assessing such claims of inequity requires detailed information about wages paid in the immediate area, and there are both legal and practical restrictions on how such information may be obtained. Many a manager has given in to the temptation to conduct a personal wage survey, calling on contacts with colleagues throughout the community to determine what other organizations are paying for the specific kinds of skills in question.

Not too many years ago—in some areas, well into the late 1980s—health care organizations freely exchanged pay scales. The U.S. Department of Justice eventually decided that not-for-profit health care organizations should be held to the same standards as other industries and began to clamp down on the free exchange of wage information—which legally constitutes an element of "price fixing" under antitrust regulations. So the department manager who solicits wage information from a colleague at another institution is technically engaging in illegal activity.

Wage surveys are permitted, but only when conducted in a particular manner. They must be done by a third-party organization (such as a membership association of hospitals or other providers) and must include a sufficient number of organizations surveyed and with data arranged in such a way that no participating institutions can be readily identified. Generally, five or six organizations are enough for an appropriate survey, provided that none can be readily identified (for example, the survey cannot have categories for "university medical centers" or "hospitals of 100 to 200 beds" if there is only one of each in the survey's area of coverage).

Rather than attempting to verify the validity of employees' claims of general inequities relative to other organizations, the department manager should take the issue to Human Resources and rely on HR to conduct the appropriate investigation.

When Interviewing Prospective Employees

Since the department manager is expected to be conversant with all the pay scales used in the department, in most organizations the manager may cite the appropriate pay range for a job during an interview. However, the manager should not attempt to make a specific financial offer during an interview. Having made a decision to offer a position to a particular applicant, the manager should collaborate with the Human Resources recruiter to determine the starting pay that will be offered, and the official offer will flow from HR to the applicant.

There are several reasons for making formal offers through Human Resources only. First, all offers of employment are extended conditionally—assuming successful reference checks and the person passing a pre-employment physical examination. Second, it is part of the Human Resources compensation task to protect the compensation system against the intrusion of inequities, which can best be accomplished only if all offers emanate from a single point. Third, some organizations' policies for determining starting-pay offers may state, for example, that someone with a given amount of experience can be offered a starting pay at a certain percentage of the pay grade. Again, this is best controlled if all offers emanate from a single point.

The department manager should of course have a voice in recommending starting pay if there is any flexibility at all in doing so. This should be done in conjunction with Human Resources, but it is always HR that extends the formal offer.

BENEFITS

The department manager should have basic benefits information available for employees, at least that information in the personnel policy and procedure manual and perhaps the employee handbook. No matter how strongly employees are urged to become familiar with their benefits, a great many of them show no interest in doing so until a specific need arises. Then when a specific need does arise, they do not proceed to read up on the benefits—rather, they choose to ask someone, usually the department manager or someone in Human Resources. This is especially true concerning health and dental insurance benefits, of which many employees remain nearly completely ignorant until a specific need emerges.

The department manager is not expected to be an expert in the interpretation of employee benefits, but the manager should be conversant enough with the benefits structure to answer employees' simpler questions and especially to know the appropriate person in HR to refer employees to for answers to benefits questions. Some areas of employee benefits can become fairly complex—for example, a sizable hospital may carry five or six different health insurance plans, each with its own hundreds of details—and questions about them are best addressed by the very few people in the organization who are versed in these details.

Flexible Benefits Plans

Flexible benefits plans, initially commonly referred to as "cafeteria" plans, proliferated through the 1980s and 1990s. It seems clear that the majority of workers prefer having some choice in benefits, and the array available to choose from is often a consideration in determining whether someone will accept employment with a particular employer.

The three benefits preferred by the majority of employees, in order of their preference, are: health insurance, pension plan, and paid vacation. However, not even these, which have for many organizations been the core of their benefits programs, are of equal importance to everyone.

Employee benefits are available in many different forms and varieties, and not all employees want or need all the same benefits. Even pension benefits, which seem ultimately to concern everyone, are not a consistent choice of all employees at all times. Often younger employees pay far less attention to pension plans, preferring more cash in hand or perhaps more paid vacation, while older employees tend to lean more toward pension benefits. Thus, choice entered benefits programs as employers endeavored to make their benefits budgets go as far as possible while giving as many employees as possible what they perceived they needed most.

It seems clear that flexibility and choice will be increasingly important features of benefits programs.

Flexible benefits plans have proven their appeal to many employees, and an increasing number of employers are offering plans that are wholly flexible or partly flexible around a small set of "core" benefits. Especially successful have been some of the programs that allow an employee to waive medical coverage (upon establishing that coverage is provided by other means, say through a spouse's employment) and apply the value of that benefit elsewhere. Also popular are plans that permit buying or selling a certain amount of vacation time by trading it off with other benefits.

A logical progression beyond flexible benefits is the use of *benefits vouchers*. These provide employees with the equivalent of a certain amount of money to apply outside of the organization as they choose, in effect spending the organization's contribution toward their benefits on what means the most to them. Vouchers have proven to be especially advantageous to some employees in this era of layoffs and downsizing; many employer-furnished benefits end when employment ends, but benefits secured externally (as with vouchers) are purchased for a certain period of time and do not necessarily end when employment ends.

Another up-and-coming approach is *voluntary benefits*. This approach allows employees to purchase certain insurance coverages and savings and retirement financial products at their place of employment. Voluntary benefits have been in use in work organizations to some extent for many years in the form of supplemental insurance programs, but the concept appears to be spreading to include some benefits formerly regarded as core benefits.

Another concept that is steadily gaining ground in benefits administration is *portable benefits*. This concept has been advanced by many as the solution to maintaining benefits for workers in this mobile society. It recognizes that individuals may work for several different organizations in the course of a normal career, and therefore may be best served by benefits that can move with them. Defined benefit plans have in many instance given way to defined contribution plans, often 401(k) plans (investments and savings) or 403(b) plans (tax-deferred annuities) that individuals can transfer with them to subsequent employers. Also addressing an aspect of benefits portability is the Health Insurance Portability and Accountability Act (HIPAA), which provides for continuity of coverage when workers change employers.

Some have predicted that the ultimate direction in benefits is toward employers offering no benefits at all other than those required by law (FICA, worker's compensation, etc.), but simply paying employees the value of the organization's benefits contribution as a part of salary and allowing them to do as they choose. This, however, would seem to be in conflict with the direction the government has established in employment legislation encouraging employers toward greater social responsibility for their employees. "No benefits other than those required by law" is exactly what a great many workers in the lower tiers of the economy presently receive—a circumstance that government has been trying to address, especially with regard to health insurance.

Statutory Benefits

A few programs that usually fall within Human Resources' areas of responsibility can be described as statutory benefits programs, in that they exist by virtue of legal requirement. Foremost among these in all states are worker's compensation and unemployment compensation, and in a number of states there is also a requirement for short-term disability compensation. The effort necessary to coordinate these programs usually falls to Human Resources, although there are implications for the department manager.

Worker's Compensation

Worker's compensation laws are in effect in all 50 states as well as in American Samoa, the District of Columbia, Guam, Puerto Rico, and the Virgin Islands. Covering both medical benefits and compensation for lost income, worker's compensation costs paid out on behalf of American employees run into the multiple billions of dollars every year.

The medical benefits paid under worker's compensation laws generally amount to full actual medical expenses. The amount of benefit paid for lost wages varies considerably from state to state, but nationwide the most common benefit paid amounts to two-third of wages up to some specified maximum. Most states place limits on both maximum and minimum, weekly benefits, the total number of weeks that benefits can be received, and the total dollar amount of benefit eligibility. Most states also provide lifetime payment for permanent disability, and some states also pay additional amounts for dependents, rehabilitation services, and other benefits.

The department manager cannot do much to influence worker's compensation costs, since the manager is one of a number of people in the organization who have separate but not well defined roles in controlling worker's compensation costs. The best approach to controlling such costs is to have an effective accident prevention program. Here the manager's role is to be constantly aware of the requirements of the program and ensure that all employees observe those requirements. Specifically, it is up to the manager to ensure that employees:

- Are thoroughly educated in safe work practices, including, in the health care setting, safe lifting techniques and safe handling of needles and other sharps. (Puncture wounds have always been a concern in health care, and back strain resulting from improper lifting remains one of the most common on-the-job injuries experienced by health care personnel.)
- Adhere to all the safety rules in place in the organization, those mandated by government as well as those established by the institution.
- Make full and appropriate use of all required safety equipment in the performance of their jobs.

In pursuing an effective accident prevention program, the manager is clearly responsible for encouraging a high level of consciousness of the need for safety among employees. In doing so it may be necessary for the manager to deal directly with employees' unsafe practices in a disciplinary manner. A violation of a safety rule is as much of a transgression as a violation of any other work rule or policy. Violators must be counseled appropriately, and if they continue to be violators they must eventually be dealt with through progressive discipline.

The department manager should also work with Human Resources in monitoring worker's compensation claims and challenging those that appear to be inappropriate. To monitor claims properly it is necessary that the manager be thorough and timely in providing all documentation that may have a bearing on a claim, that is, all necessary incident reports and accident reports should be provided as soon as possible after the fact and should be clear and detailed.

Questions will often arise about whether a particular injury occurred during working time or on the institution's property, and it may be necessary to take steps to determine whether worker's compensation is appropriate or whether the case is more likely to fall under short-term disability as an off-the-job occurrence. Employees will sometimes report off-the-job accidents as occurring on the job, especially in those states and those organizations where there is no short-term disability benefit or where worker's compensation benefits are more generous than short-term disability benefits. After an injured employee's personal physician, the employee's supervisor is often the next most important person in determining whether a given occurrence legitimately falls under worker's compensation.

Unemployment Compensation

The Social Security Act of 1935 made the individual states responsible for their own unemployment compensation insurance programs. A federal tax was imposed on employers, but most of this tax could be offset by state taxes. All programs were to be controlled at state level.

Unemployment insurance programs are in effect in all 50 states plus the District of Columbia and Puerto Rico. These programs are continually undergoing change, with the majority of these changes resulting in increased benefits to employees and increased costs to employers.

Although differences exist throughout the country, employers are generally subject to experience rating; that is, they are taxed according to their past records, so an employer that decreases its unemployment claims by employees will also decrease its unemployment tax bill. The majority of business organizations, and virtually all profit-making businesses, are taxed directly using experience-based rates established by the various states. However, in a number of states, not-for-profit organizations, including most health care organizations, pay for their unemployment on a dollar-for-dollar basis rather than paying a tax based on a percentage of payroll; that is, such organizations pay their actual unemployment costs as they are incurred.

Since unemployment compensation is intended to make up for wages lost due to periods of unemployment beyond the employee's control, unemployment compensation is not ordinarily made available to people who voluntarily resign their employment or who are discharged for cause. Rather, unemployment compensation is intended primarily for employees who are laid off through no fault of their own or who otherwise find that their services are no longer required. Individuals who have been dismissed due to their apparent inability to meet the requirements of their positions also generally qualify for unemployment compensation. In a few states, employees who are on strike can receive unemployment compensation after a specified waiting period (six or more weeks from the start of the strike).

To the extent that it might be possible for the department manager to influence certain kinds of employee turnover, it is possible for the manager to have an effect on the organization's unemployment compensation costs. Following are some guidelines for the manager's consideration:

- Care and thoroughness in hiring will help limit the likelihood of acquiring an employee who may turn out to be unable to do the job. It is not possible to refine the hiring process to the point where one will always know that the right choice is being made; nevertheless, if the manager sticks to normal minimum education and experience requirements and does not rush a decision based on insufficient information or an insufficient number of candidates, it may be possible to head off performance problems before they begin. In the process of heading off potential performance problems, the manager will also be avoiding potential unemployment costs.

- Regarding hiring, orientation, and especially the application of disciplinary action, the manager should scrupulously follow all of the organization's policies and all applicable legal processes. Disciplinary actions, especially those taken in a series that could eventually result in termination, are especially important. All such actions need to be thoroughly documented and should be taken strictly in accordance with policy and with EEO guidelines. Since many non-legitimate claims for unemployment compensation are made, it is frequently necessary to use records of disciplinary actions to refute such claims. Also, since the acknowledged primary purpose of disciplinary action is correction of behavior, it is often necessary to produce documentation of a series of related actions to demonstrate that an employee had the opportunity to correct the errant behavior but failed to do so.

- If it is at all possible, the manager should act to remove a substandard performer during the probationary period. The organization's probationary period may be too short a time in which to be able to make a definite decision concerning an employee's ability, especially the ability of an apparently marginal employee. However, the probationary period is often sufficient to give the manager a strong indication of where the employee is heading. Separation for performance-related reasons is usually easier to justify outside of the organization if it occurs by the expiration of an understood probationary period. Also, because an institution's unemployment costs are related to the length of time an employee has worked for that organization, separation by the end of the probationary period reduces the organization's cost exposure.

- Working in conjunction with Human Resources, the manager should challenge all unemployment claims that appear inappropriate. Many people automatically file for unemployment regardless of why or how they left their positions; they have nothing to lose by trying. Many will state their reasons for termination clearly in their favor, and it then becomes necessary for the organization to dispute such claims to avoid unemployment costs. If a claim goes undisputed, the employee, deserving or not, will automatically collect unemployment compensation. Thus, every effort should be made to dispute each inappropriate claim.

- The manager should consider the use of temporary help when it is known that certain requirements will be of short duration. Hiring a regular employee to cover a given need and laying off the person when the need has passed automatically creates exposure to unemployment costs. The use of temporary help, engaged specifically for certain tasks or for known brief periods of time, will avoid such costs. In most parts of the country it requires six months (26 weeks) of work for a single employee to move the organization to the point of maximum exposure to unemployment costs, so any need of less than six months that can be covered by temporary help reduces the organization's exposure to unemployment costs.

Short-Term Disability

Unlike worker's compensation and unemployment compensation, which are statutory requirements throughout the country, short-term disability (DBL) is not a widespread legal requirement. However, when coverage is in place by virtue of the employer's choice rather than by requirement of law, it nevertheless requires the same level of conscientious attention to cost control.

Most organizations are experience-rated regarding disability. Any year's actual experience—that is, the claims actually paid—is directly reflected in the next year's premium rates. Therefore, most organizations pay dollar-for-dollar; they eventually pay the total actual costs of all claims, plus administrative expenses.

The single action that can have the greatest impact on the organization's disability costs overall is a corporate decision to go with self-insurance, coupled with a comprehensive employee health and safety program. At the level of the individual department, the manager can:

- Pass along to employees information the organization may supply concerning personal health and safety in general and certain hazards or illnesses in particular
- Urge employees to take advantage of the annual physical examinations or health assessments that many organizations offer, and always be prepared to refer employees to the employee health office when questions arise or problems become apparent
- Scrupulously fulfill all departmental responsibilities in following disability procedures, ensuring that all necessary forms are completed thoroughly and in a timely fashion.

THE EMPLOYMENT PROCESS

One dimension of the employment process that may be largely invisible to the department manager is the extent to which Human Resources may have to go to secure candidates who meet the job's minimum stated requirements. How much has to happen behind the scenes depends on the position for which recruiting is being done and the general state of the employment market. If many people are seeking work, it is usually not a significant task for HR to come up with five or six viable candidates for most entry-level positions or perhaps even several candidates for the majority of somewhat specialized positions. Regardless of the general state of the employment market, however, it can be an entirely different matter locating candidates in occupations that may be in short supply.

A number of health care occupations have experienced shortages, some chronic, and at times HR has undoubtedly been fortunate to find just one or two candidates for particular openings. Such shortages have been experienced, for example, with registered pharmacists, physical therapists, occupational therapists, and physician assistants. From the manager's perspective it is best to have a choice of several viable candidates immediately after the position opens. However, the practicalities of supply can dictate that there may not be as many to choose from as one might prefer, and these might not be immediately available.

The department manager undoubtedly sees more than just the tip of the iceberg as far as the recruiting process is concerned, and most of what can be said about the Human Resources role versus the department manager's role has been covered in earlier chapters. It is mentioned here only as a reminder that once the manager conveys a hiring decision to Human Resources, a number of activities not visible to the manager can affect a new employee's starting date.

The most time-consuming steps involved in getting a new employee cleared and on board are usually checking employment references and getting the person through a pre-employment physical examination. Reference checking can require two or three days, although this is being done more quickly all the time thanks to technology (e.g., fax machines). The pre-employment physical examination means securing an appointment, having the exam done, and awaiting the results that clear the person to begin work. If the organization is operating in a state in which a health care employee is not permitted to start work without the physical exam, little can be done to expedite the process.

Although a new employee cannot begin the day the hiring decision is made, he or she can usually be completely cleared in one work week. Should a new hire be employed elsewhere and need to work out a standard two-week notice, the individual should be completely cleared to begin work by the time that notice period is satisfied.

PERFORMANCE APPRAISAL

Often all the department manager seems to see and hear about performance appraisal are evaluations to be done, timetables for completion, and "nagging" reminders about staying on schedule (see Chapter 10, Performance Appraisal: The Never-Ending Task).

At its best, performance appraisal is a valuable employee development mechanism; at its worst, it is a bureaucratic exercise required by accreditation and regulatory agencies. But whichever end of the scale it tends toward in any particular organization, it is a requirement and Human Resources is usually charged with making certain it happens according to a specific process and timetable. In attending to performance appraisal requirements, HR will ordinarily:

- Keep the appraisal form and process current, updating the procedure as necessary and disseminating changes
- Provide evaluator training, both initial training for first-time evaluators and annual refresher training for all others as necessary
- Arrange for the preparation and distribution of appraisal forms, instructions, and schedules at the proper time
- Remain available to address questions raised by evaluators and employees
- Follow up with department managers to ensure timely completion of appraisals
- Collect and audit appraisals and follow up on missing information
- Arrange for tabulation of appraisals and preparation of summary information for executive management and for calculation of merit increases (if using a pay-for-performance system)
- File completed appraisals in employees' personnel files.

LEGAL ACTIONS

Chapter 14, See You in Court: Involvement in Legal Action, has essentially provided a look at most of the iceberg as far as the department manager's involvement in legal actions is concerned. Although the focus of Chapter 14 was primarily employment-related actions, many of the same requirements on the manager will prevail for actions involving malpractice charges or charges arising from general liability.

From the department manager's perspective, involvement in a legal action may take the form of brief periods of extremely intense, perhaps overly demanding activity, interspersed with lengthy stretches of little or no visible activity. The following are some guidelines for the department manager who may become involved in a legal action against the organization:

- Be patient. Because of attorneys' schedules, court calendars, official waiting times, and other considerations, legal actions take time to resolve. There is little point in allowing the suspense of a situation to hang heavily over your head when the timing of events lies well beyond an individual's control.

- Accept the normal sequence of events. During long, seemingly quiet periods, nothing at all may be happening. On the other hand, very much that does not involve the manager may be happening—such as motions, depositions of various individuals, and settlement conferences. The pace toward resolution invariably seems slow, so once again the best recourse is to accept that which cannot be controlled.
- Don't be overly concerned about the possibility that you will be called for deposition or trial testimony. Plenty of expert preparation and support will be provided.
- Accept the inevitable. If you are named in a charge or otherwise summoned in the case, there is no way to avoid appearing. Even resigning your employment will not erase the legal obligation.
- Write only what it is necessary to write, and always do so objectively and without personal bias or name-calling. Complete all forms thoroughly, with special attention to dates and signatures.
- Remain sensitive to the implications of the case in day-to-day dealings with employees, remaining mindful that words as well as actions can cause problems.
- Even in response to direct questioning, do not discuss an open case with others in the organization except for those few who are actively managing involvement (case coordinator, etc.). Avoid the temptation to make predictions concerning the eventual outcome.

EXTERNAL AGENCY INVESTIGATIONS

A considerable amount of time is generally spent, much of it by Human Resources staff, relating with representatives of various government agencies. The more commonly encountered agencies are:

- *Equal Employment Opportunity Commission (EEOC) and the State Division of Human Rights (DHR).* These two agencies deal with allegations of employment discrimination. To file a complaint with one is essentially to file with both; in many states a complaint reaching EEOC first is automatically referred to DHR for initial processing. These agencies' initial point of contact in the organization is usually Human Resources, and it is ordinarily HR that will go through the process of gathering the requested information and formally responding to the complaint. The manager of the complaining employee's department will often be contacted for information to help in developing the organization's response, and the manager will likely be interviewed during investigation of the complaint.

- *Occupational Safely and Health Administration (OSHA).* On no particular schedule or set frequency, this agency may send representatives to perform routine surveys of safety practices or to investigate specific complaints they have received concerning allegations of unsafe practices. Human Resources is often the OSHA point of contact in the organization, but the contact may also be someone in Administration or perhaps a designated risk manager or safety manager. Plant engineering may also be involved since so many safety issues involve the physical plant. The manager of a department where a possible unsafe practice is observed or alleged can expect to become involved.

- *State Employment Service.* Human Resources is heavily involved in every claim for unemployment compensation. Since an employee's level of compensation is based on earnings, earnings information must be provided. Human Resources must also supply the reason for termination and must indicate whether the claim will be protested or not. A protested claim usually results in a hearing before an administrative law judge, and a hearing usually involves the former employee's immediate supervisor as well as a Human Resources representative.

- *Immigration and Naturalization Service (INS).* Investigators from the INS will periodically arrive in Human Resources to audit personnel files for the presence and accurate completion of the required I-9 forms. Ordinarily the department manager will have no involvement in an I-9 audit except possibly as the channel for an I-9–related question from HR to an employee. Occasionally, however, INS investigators will come looking into specific individuals' immigration status, and such investigations could mean questions for the department manager.

- *Department of Labor (DOL).* The Department of Labor monitors compliance with wage-and-hour laws. Since there are both state and federal wage-and-hour laws, the organization may occasionally be visited by state or federal DOL representatives. Their interest may simply be a routine audit of certain wage payment practices—the proper payment of overtime seems to be a special interest of theirs—or an investigation of certain employment practices (e.g., compliance with child labor laws). DOL investigators will on occasion arrive because someone has registered a complaint alleging some irregularity in wage payment. The DOL's primary points of contact in the organization will ordinarily be Human Resources and Payroll, but department managers can become involved in providing information needed in determining, for example, whether an employee is properly classified (as exempt or nonexempt) or whether time worked has been appropriately reported.

No one is particularly fond of having their daily routine disrupted by the arrival of representatives of an external agency, especially since many such visits are seen as indicating trouble of some kind. However, such contacts are inevitable, so your Human Resources department should regard all such external agency inquiries as opportunities to review various practices for possible violations and determine how these practices might be improved. Even though the occasional external investigator can come across as unnecessarily forceful, it accomplishes nothing for HR personnel or others to become defensive or uncooperative.

A considerable part of the Human Resources role regarding external agencies is to know the law as well as the agency's guidelines and procedures. In looking into a specific complaint internally, HR should first try to determine whether it is valid, and if so should recommend corrective action in addition to formulating the organization's response to the agency. There is surely no gain in resisting a complaint if the organization appears to be in the wrong. However, HR professionals are usually well aware that an investigator who is acting on an individual's complaint has heard only one side of the story.

Unless the particular complaint to be addressed is a discrimination charge (i.e., from EEOC or DHR) that cannot be disposed of at an early stage, Human Resources is usually able to keep the department manager's involvement with external agency representatives to a minimum.

Discussion Points

1. Explain, with several examples, what is meant by the term *statutory benefits*.

2. Explain why the department manager should be thoroughly conversant with the pay scales appropriate to the department but refrain from making specific pay offers to potential employees.

3. You are approached by an employee who complains that he is being paid less than another employee who is doing the same work. Discuss how you would respond and what you would do.

4. Discuss why the department manager should avoid trying to compare employee pay scales with those of other organizations.

5. Consider what your initial reaction should be if, first thing Monday morning, a representative of an external regulatory organization walks into your department and declares, "I'm here to audit your activity."

6. Explain how you, as department manager, should proceed if you believe you have uncovered a severe shortcoming of the performance appraisal process as it applies to a particular group of your employees.

7. Discuss how you will respond to an employee who asks, "What's the difference between a defined benefit pension plan and a defined contribution plan, and which do we have here?"

8. Explain why there is increasing interest in and attention to *portable benefits*, in health care and elsewhere.

9. Describe what you believe to be the department manager's primary role in attempting to control worker's compensation costs.

10. Provide at least three reasons why it is ordinarily not possible to offer an applicant a job today and have the person begin work tomorrow.

11. There is sometimes disagreement concerning whether a particular instance of time lost due to injury or illness should be considered under worker's compensation (job-related) or short-term disability (not job-related). Explain why the distinction is important, keeping in mind that the employer ultimately pays both.

12. Describe what you believe the department manager's role should be in controlling the cost of unemployment compensation.

CHAPTER 18

Keeping Human Resources on Its Toes

This chapter—

- Describes the characteristics of an effective Human Resources department
- Advises department managers to adopt a proactive approach with Human Resources, suggesting how to approach HR in a number of areas of concern
- Suggests where the changing shape of Human Resources may be taking this function during the coming years
- Suggests how top management can strengthen the value and effectiveness of the Human Resources function.

THE EFFECTIVE HUMAN RESOURCES DEPARTMENT

The department manager will ordinarily have sufficient contact with Human Resources to be able to draw some conclusions concerning its effectiveness. In viewing an effective Human Resources department, the department manager should see:

- Visible concern for people as valued assets and as individuals rather than as disposable commodities
- Visible top management support for Human Resources and its programs, with inclusion of HR management on the organization's administrative team
- A compensation structure that is competitive within the industry's local region and that recognizes and rewards performance

- A similarly competitive benefits structure that can accommodate a variety of employee needs
- Effective and constructively focused training and development activities
- Policies that foster the opportunity for promotion and growth within the organization
- Open and honest communication that allows employees to feel included and to know what is happening within the organization
- The ability to retain employees, as exhibited by an employee turnover rate less than the regional average for the industry
- An atmosphere in which employee participation is encouraged and employee input is valued.

Visible weaknesses in any of these areas should be taken as signs of needed improvement. Neither department management nor executive management should be hesitant to bring apparent weaknesses to the attention of HR management. HR management may not be able to fix some problems—top management support may not be extended, money may not be available, or there may be external obstacles beyond their control—but HR management will undoubtedly be able to take some positive steps to improve effectiveness once a need has been pointed out.

BE PROACTIVE WITH YOUR HUMAN RESOURCES DEPARTMENT

Every department manager has occasional or even frequent needs that can be addressed entirely or in part by the Human Resources department—but only if HR is made aware of the nature of the needs and the extent of the assistance required. As a department manager in occasional need of assistance, do not wait for Human Resources to figure out your needs and offer help. Rather, be proactive—put Human Resources on the spot, and challenge HR to provide needed assistance.

Once you ascertain that your need falls within HR's sphere of responsibility, find out who in Human Resources is most likely to address your kind of issue, and follow up with the appropriate person. Thoroughly explain what you need, negotiate agreement with HR, including a reasonable deadline, and hold HR to that deadline. As you should in dealing with anyone, whether an employee in your own department or someone from another area, if a reasonable deadline arrives and there has been no response, actively follow up. It is fully as essential in dealing with HR as with anyone else to never allow a deadline of any kind to pass unanswered without following up.

Involve HR in Compensation Questions

Always bring Human Resources into the process of resolving wage complaints, especially those involving scale inequities both real and perceived. Specific paycheck inquiries, that is, questions about errors on an employee's paycheck, can be addressed either by Human Resources or by the payroll section of Finance, depending on the organization's payroll system.

Get Answers for Employees

When an employee has a question that involves HR matters that you cannot answer yourself, take the issue to Human Resources. Do not always simply *send* the employee to HR; go there yourself. In doing so you will better prepare yourself to respond to future employee questions, and at the same time you will be demonstrating to both the employee and HR that you are interested in the employee's concerns.

Address Recruitment Issues

When you are provided with applications and resumes to review for possible interviews, review them promptly and get them back to HR with your interview preferences. In turning these around promptly, you are serving two important purposes: (1) you are serving your needs in speeding up the process of arranging interviews, and (2) you are keeping the ball in HR's court and making it necessary for HR to respond to you. This issue surfaces time and again in strained relations between HR and the departments: A manager complains to higher-ups that HR is slow in providing interview prospects, while HR in turn complains that the manager has been sitting on a pile of applications for weeks without response.

When dealing with HR recruiters in attempting to fill a position, if you feel that there are no genuinely appropriate candidates in the five or six that you have been sent to interview, do not hesitate to request more. However, resist the temptation to go overboard in looking for the "perfect" candidate. As noted in Chapter 6, The Manager and the Recruiting Process, if Human Resources is doing the job it ought to be doing, the five or six applicants provided for interview will all meet the stated minimum qualifications for the position. If it is an entry-level position, any one of these five or six could probably do the job; the selection process will then revolve around the assessment of how well each of these applicants might fit into the group. Some managers show a tendency to keep looking for the "perfect" candidate, someone who fits ideally into the group and who can hit the ground running at 100 percent productivity with little or no training—in other words, the candidate who under most circumstances does not exist.

When dealing with an HR recruiter in filling a position, once you have made your tentative selection and agreed with HR on a tentative offer, stay in close contact with the recruiter concerning the status of reference checking, the scheduling of a pre-employment physical examination, and other pre-employment concerns. Without making a nuisance of yourself—a call each day or two should suffice—this indication of your active interest should serve to help keep the process moving.

Insist on Current Job Descriptions

Keep your department's job descriptions up to date, and make certain that Human Resources keeps current in evaluating your department's jobs to ensure they are correctly graded and associated with the proper pay scales. Job descriptions should be reviewed whenever there is a change in method, procedure, or equipment that affects the performance of the job. A job description should be updated at the time the changes are effective; it should not be left until someone suddenly realizes that an up-to-date job description is needed for recruiting or performance appraisal or for some other immediate purpose.

Use HR for Support on Disciplinary Actions

Make appropriate use of HR assistance concerning disciplinary actions. Human Resources does not actually perform disciplinary actions and should never be expected to do so (except within the HR department itself), but HR should always be expected to be available for guidance regarding the consistency, appropriateness, and legality of disciplinary actions. Every disciplinary action of any consequence should be reviewed with HR before it is finalized and delivered, and the department manager should unfailingly go to HR for advice and should expect to receive it. The ultimate decision in a disciplinary action will likely reside with you, the department manager, but never allow Human Resources to avoid its responsibility for providing specific guidance.

Ask Human Resources if there is a system in place for invalidating or removing past disciplinary actions that are in employees' personnel files. There should be an agreed-upon time limit following which, if there are no additional related infractions, an employee can expect that a once-valid warning document will no longer officially exist. One facility's system, for example, calls for a written warning to be invalidated 22 months after it is issued if no additional related infractions have occurred during that time. A regular purge of personnel files for this purpose is impractical, but whenever a particular file is reviewed or audited and an action older than 22 months is found, it is removed to a separate, central file (none are destroyed, however, in case one should ever become pertinent to a future legal action). The point of invalidating older warnings, of course, is that an infraction should not be held against an employee permanently if correction has been accomplished and maintained for a reasonable period of time.

Keep HR Moving on Performance Appraisals As Necessary

Especially if your organization's system calls for anniversary date appraisals, keep track of scheduled review dates for your department's employees. Be prepared to follow up with HR if appraisal forms and schedules are not forthcoming when you believe they should be. Although it is most likely HR's responsibility to distribute appraisal schedules and forms at certain times, HR can be fully as subject to laxity or error as anyone else. One might be tempted to quietly look the other way if the possibly dreaded appraisal task is not forthcoming when it is expected, but this simply puts the task under greater time pressure when it does occur. If you need to convey a reminder to HR so you can keep your appraisals on schedule, do so.

Should Human Resources neglect to periodically offer refresher training in performance appraisal, ask for it. Every year or so, and whenever there are changes in the appraisal instrument, refresher training in the use of the system should be provided. If HR is not proactive in offering such training, the department managers should push for it. Also, at some time following each full appraisal cycle, usually annually, follow up with HR to request appraisal history and statistics—

specifically, what the range and average of scores were for your department and for the organization as a whole.

Use Human Resources to Clip "the Grapevine"

One way or another, the organization's informal, socially based communication network—otherwise known as the grapevine—will prevail. It can make employees feel threatened and helpless; it can make managers feel frustrated and embarrassed; it can spread bad news, good news, truth, untruth, and any manner of speculation often faster than most legitimate means of communication; and it can impede and impair effective management decision-making. But it cannot be eradicated.

The Human Resources department is the focus of much employee communication. Most HR practitioners are in a position to know much of what is accurate and to hear quickly what is being reported on the grapevine; they have long known that the grapevine, although it often distorts information, can carry information extremely rapidly. As a result, many HR professionals believe that the key concern in addressing the grapevine is not trying to muzzle it or eliminate it but to manage it.

The surest way of managing the grapevine is to give it something accurate to carry. Probably one of the greatest communication mistakes a manager can make upon hearing something from the "rumor mill" is to pass it along without verification or correction.

Open, honest, free-flowing organizational communication will serve to hold the grapevine's appeal to a minimum. The more employees feel left out, they more they feel that information is withheld from them, the more they will speculate and the more they will share their speculations with others. This of course applies to all employees organization-wide, but it also applies to the employees within a department. The department manager who is generally uncommunicative is leaving the employees to "fill in the gaps" in their information by talking with each other and with employees from other departments. The less continuing contact the manager has with the employees, the more likely these employees are to seek information from other employees.

In viewing the grapevine from the individual department perspective, the department manager should:

- Always remember that an effective, continuing relationship with each employee is one of the best possible defenses against unwarranted speculation. You should seek to achieve a level of rapport with employees such that upon hearing a rumor the first thing they do is check it out with you.

- When uncertainty prevails and tensions are running high over some supposedly upcoming dramatic event—merger, affiliation, new CEO—and you feel you can say nothing because you know nothing of substance, say it anyway. In other words, keep talking with your employees, even if the best you can say is "I know no more than you do," "I'm trying to find out for you," or "I'll let you know as soon as I hear." Even when you have nothing significant to pass along, stay in touch with employees.
- When a grapevine story reaches you and you know it to be incorrect, pass along the correct information. Information will travel the grapevine regardless of what you do, so you might as well give it something correct to carry when possible.
- Since a great many rumors that travel the grapevine have Human Resources implications (pay, benefits, employment, restructuring, etc.) and since HR is the focal point of much official employee communication, take all significant rumors to Human Resources. Human Resources is in the best position to issue organization-wide disclaimers when necessary, and HR can often give you the correct information to carry back to your employees.

Take Training Needs to HR

Unless there is a separate education department to address training needs, go to Human Resources with any training needs that you cannot completely and competently fill within your own department. HR will be able to provide some kinds of training directly, or HR may be able to broker such training by putting you in touch with those who can supply what is needed.

Provide Current Information to HR

The professionals in the Human Resources department will ordinarily be doing the best they can to remain current in fulfilling the needs of the line departments. To do so, however, HR needs to hear regularly from the department managers concerning what can be done to best serve present and emerging needs. Do not expect Human Resources to second-guess your needs, but rather let HR know, for example:

- What policies and procedures you believe may need to be revisited for possible revision based on changing conditions in department operations
- Specific recommendations you can make for recruiting and retaining the particular skills used in your department
- The kinds of complaints—or compliments—you may be hearing from employees concerning the organization's policies
- Any employee feedback that may reflect employee attitudes toward pay, benefits, and other conditions of employment.

Encourage Human Resources to Prove Its Worth

Human Resources services are often viewed as largely "soft" and thus not effectively measured. However, there are many ways to measure HR effectiveness. For example, it is possible to examine:

- Key indicators concerning employment activity, such as average cost per hire and average time required to fill a position
- Employee retention and other issues, by addressing turnover by organization, department, or job title, and by month, quarter, or year
- HR cost as a percentage of total expenses or staffing as a ratio of HR staff to total number of employees
- The effectiveness of training, as measured by pre-training and post-training testing and by observable behavior change.

Encourage Human Resources to establish baselines for measuring its own performance. Compare these baselines with industry benchmarks and use them for HR's comparisons with itself from year to year or period to period. Overall, encourage both the measurement of Human Resources performance and the visibility of the results.

FUTURE DIRECTIONS FOR HUMAN RESOURCES

No one knows for certain what the future will bring. Based on experiences of the recent past and present trends and signs, however, we can perhaps advance a few possibilities for what the future may hold for the Human Resources department in the health care organization.

In some critical dimensions the Human Resources function will probably increase in importance, but at the same time it may continue to shrink in terms of numbers of HR staff. If the health care organization is to increase productivity, compete successfully, and survive financially, it must continue to improve the effectiveness with which it uses its people—its human resources.

We will likely see a continued increase in the outsourcing of routine HR functions, but also increasing concern with strategic issues and policy matters. Human Resources may see more centralization of policy-making and administration of programs, yet more decentralization in application as centralized HR functions serve a growing number of multi-facility health systems.

We will probably experience the steadily increasing importance of management development as line managers assume more responsibility and a broader span of control. At the same time, however, service in this area will lag for economic reasons as non-clinical education continues to be an early budget-cutting target in most economically strapped organizations.

Human Resources will likely experience increased automation in creating and maintaining records and eventually the integration of personnel records with data from other sources.

In matters of compensation we will likely experience the increasing use of merit-based (pay-for-performance) systems and a corresponding decline in automatic time-based or "cost-of-living" increases.

In matters of benefits we will experience the broader proliferation of programs that offer employee choice.

Health care organizations will also likely be paying closer attention to employee attitudes in an effort to stay closer to employees and learn how to get them more interested and involved.

There may well be a renewed emphasis on productivity enhancement programs as health care continues trying to do more with less and provide quality service with constrained resources.

Finally, we will likely experience increasing concern for organizational values and for the culture of the organization, with ongoing attention to the organization's mission, vision, and goals.

FOR TOP MANAGEMENT'S CONSIDERATION

One of the most important questions top management can ask concerning Human Resources is: Do we have essentially a reactionary HR department—a crisis occurs, then HR acts? In other words, is there insufficient systematic assessment of the organization's needs to identify potential problems in advance? Executive management is urged to think more long-term regarding HR policy and direction if it is not already doing so.

Human Resource professionals are best used as internal consultants to management, involved in strategic planning and serving as part of the executive team, rather than being considered simply a resource to call on when a crisis seems to have HR implications.

Top management should insist on linking plans for recruitment, retention, training and development, performance appraisal, and compensation and benefits, etc., to the organization's overall strategies. Human Resources planning should be an integral part of the organization's strategic planning process, with management insisting on close cooperation between HR planning and corporate planning.

Top management should insist on the involvement of both Human Resources professionals and line managers in designing HR programs to meet the organization's real needs, and should always insist on the involvement of line managers to the maximum extent possible in implementing HR programs.

Overall the way for top management to get the best from the organization's Human Resources department is to insist on proactive Human Resources management while providing visible support for the HR function.

HR EXISTS TO WORK FOR YOU—SEE THAT IT HAPPENS

Human Resources exists in large part for both the individual and the organization. The Human Resources department is there to:

- Protect the rights of the individual employee—including you, the department manager—not simply because there are laws requiring the organization to do so, but because safeguarding the rights of the individual is the right thing to do
- Protect the organization from certain forms of legal risk, or at least minimize exposure to legal risk.

Human Resources means personnel, and personnel means people. Thus, every manager of people is a manager of human resources. The department called Human Resources is a staff support activity that exists to provide service that enhances the efficient functioning of the organization. In your dealings with Human Resources, make certain that you and your department's employees receive all the attention you deserve. In fact, insist on it.

Discussion Points

1. Explain why even a well-functioning, well-intended Human Resources Department may have to be "pushed" occasionally to ensure that it operates proactively in all respects.
2. From either your experience or a hypothetical situation, describe a significant shortcoming in a Human Resources Department's services and recommend how that shortcoming could be eliminated.
3. Explain why "Go talk to Human Resources" is not always the appropriate response to an employee's HR-related question.
4. From either your experience or by hypothesizing, identify a major area of specific need for your department and describe how Human Resources can best address that need.
5. Consider why it might be necessary for the department manager to remind Human Resources to keep the performance appraisal process moving, instead of Human Resources reminding the manager.
6. Discuss why many organizations require that significant disciplinary actions be cleared with Human Resources before implementation.
7. Explain what the department manager can do to ensure that Human Resources keeps the organization's job descriptions current and complete.
8. Explain how the Human Resources Department can assist department managers with employee communication needs, specifically addressing how HR can help control rumors.
9. Discuss why you should insist that Human Resources provide statistics of HR activity such as turnover, cost per hire, average time to fill a position, etc.
10. Consider why the individual department manager should have any interest in narrowing the occasional credibility gap between Human Resources and the line departments. Shouldn't this be solely HR's concern?

Index